Family–School Success for Children with ADHD

The Guilford Practical Intervention in the Schools Series

Kenneth W. Merrell, Founding Editor
Sandra M. Chafouleas, Series Editor

www.guilford.com/practical

This series presents the most reader-friendly resources available in key areas of evidence-based practice in school settings. Practitioners will find trustworthy guides on effective behavioral, mental health, and academic interventions, and assessment and measurement approaches. Covering all aspects of planning, implementing, and evaluating high-quality services for students, books in the series are carefully crafted for everyday utility. Features include ready-to-use reproducibles, appealing visual elements, and an oversized format. Recent titles have Web pages where purchasers can download and print the reproducible materials.

Recent Volumes

Child and Adolescent Suicidal Behavior, Second Edition:
School-Based Prevention, Assessment, and Intervention
David N. Miller

School Supports for Students in Military Families
Pamela Fenning

Safe and Healthy Schools, Second Edition: Practical Prevention Strategies
Jeffrey R. Sprague and Hill M. Walker

Clinical Interviews for Children and Adolescents, Third Edition:
Assessment to Intervention
Stephanie H. McConaughy and Sara A. Whitcomb

Executive Function Skills in the Classroom:
Overcoming Barriers, Building Strategies
Laurie Faith, Carol-Anne Bush, and Peg Dawson

The RTI Approach to Evaluating Learning Disabilities,
Second Edition
*Joseph F. Kovaleski, Amanda M. VanDerHeyden, Timothy J. Runge,
Perry A. Zirkel, and Edward S. Shapiro*

Effective Bullying Prevention: A Comprehensive Schoolwide Approach
Adam Collins and Jason Harlacher

Social Justice in Schools: A Framework for Equity in Education
Charles A. Barrett

Coaching Students with Executive Skills Challenges, Second Edition
Peg Dawson and Richard Guare

Social, Emotional, and Behavioral Supports in Schools:
Linking Assessment to Tier 2 Intervention
Sara C. McDaniel, Allison L. Bruhn, and Sara Estrapala

Family–School Success for Children with ADHD: A Guide for Intervention
Thomas J. Power, Jennifer A. Mautone, and Stephen L. Soffer

Family–School Success for Children with ADHD

A Guide for Intervention

**THOMAS J. POWER
JENNIFER A. MAUTONE
STEPHEN L. SOFFER**

THE GUILFORD PRESS
New York   London

Copyright © 2024 The Guilford Press
A Division of Guilford Publications, Inc.
370 Seventh Avenue, Suite 1200, New York, NY 10001
www.guilford.com

All rights reserved

Except as indicated, no part of this book may be reproduced, translated, stored in a retrieval system, or transmitted, in any form or by any means, electronic, mechanical, photocopying, microfilming, recording, or otherwise, without written permission from the publisher.

Printed in the United States of America

This book is printed on acid-free paper.

Last digit is print number: 9   8   7   6   5   4   3   2   1

LIMITED DUPLICATION LICENSE

These materials are intended for use only by qualified professionals.

The publisher grants to individual purchasers of this book nonassignable permission to reproduce all materials for which photocopying permission is specifically granted in a footnote. This license is limited to you, the individual purchaser, for personal use or use with students. This license does not grant the right to reproduce these materials for resale, redistribution, electronic display, or any other purposes (including but not limited to books, pamphlets, articles, video or audio recordings, blogs, file-sharing sites, internet or intranet sites, and handouts or slides for lectures, workshops, or webinars, whether or not a fee is charged). Permission to reproduce these materials for these and any other purposes must be obtained in writing from the Permissions Department of Guilford Publications.

The authors have checked with sources believed to be reliable in their efforts to provide information that is complete and generally in accord with the standards of practice that are accepted at the time of publication. However, in view of the possibility of human error or changes in behavioral, mental health, or medical sciences, neither the authors, nor the editor and publisher, nor any other party who has been involved in the preparation or publication of this work warrants that the information contained herein is in every respect accurate or complete, and they are not responsible for any errors or omissions or the results obtained from the use of such information. Readers are encouraged to confirm the information contained in this book with other sources.

Library of Congress Cataloging-in-Publication Data

Names: Power, Thomas J., author. | Mautone, Jennifer A., author. | Soffer, Stephen L., author.
Title: Family–school success for children with ADHD : a guide for intervention / Thomas J. Power, Jennifer A. Mautone, Stephen L. Soffer.
Description: New York : The Guilford Press, 2024. | Series: The Guilford practical intervention in the schools series | Includes bibliographical references and index.
Identifiers: LCCN 2023055961 | ISBN 9781462554362 (paperback) | ISBN 9781462554379 (hardcover)
Subjects: LCSH: Attention-deficit-disordered children—Education. | Attention-deficit-disordered children—Family relationships. | Attention-deficit hyperactivity disorder—Treatment. | Education—Parent participation. | Home and school. | BISAC: PSYCHOLOGY / Psychopathology / Attention-Deficit Disorder (ADD-ADHD) | EDUCATION / Counseling / General
Classification: LCC LC4713.2 .P689 2024 | DDC 371.94—dc23/eng/20231229
LC record available at *https://lccn.loc.gov/2023055961*

TJP: *To the many, many trainees who have re-created FSS over the years and made me a better clinician and researcher*

JAM: *To my parents, Ann and Dennis, and to John, Matthew, and Evan, for providing endless support and laughter throughout all of life's adventures*

SLS: *To Robyn, Zach, Amber, Will, and Forrest—you are my motivation to be a little better each day as a parent, partner, and person— and to my mother, Elaine, for sparking my love of science*

About the Authors

Thomas J. Power, PhD, ABPP, is Professor of School Psychology in Pediatrics and Psychiatry at the Perelman School of Medicine at the University of Pennsylvania and Distinguished Endowed Chair in the Department of Pediatrics at Children's Hospital of Philadelphia (CHOP). Dr. Power has been Director of the Center for Management of ADHD at CHOP since 1999. He spent many years providing services to children and families coping with attention-deficit/hyperactivity disorder (ADHD) and has been dedicated to interprofessional training and intervention research throughout his career. Dr. Power is a past editor of *School Psychology Review* and was a member of the Society for Developmental and Behavioral Pediatrics committee that prepared the Clinical Practice Guideline for the Assessment and Treatment of Children and Adolescents with Complex ADHD.

Jennifer A. Mautone, PhD, ABPP, is Associate Professor of School Psychology in Psychiatry at the Perelman School of Medicine at the University of Pennsylvania and Director of Primary Care Behavioral Health Research in the Department of Child and Adolescent Psychiatry and Behavioral Sciences at CHOP. Dr. Mautone served as founding Co-Director of Healthy Minds, Healthy Kids, the integrated behavioral health in primary care program at CHOP. Her research and clinical practice focus on improving connections between systems of care (for example, families, schools, health systems) and increasing equitable access to and utilization of high-quality, culturally responsive behavioral health services for children and adolescents. Dr. Mautone has published over 50 peer-reviewed papers in scientific journals.

Stephen L. Soffer, PhD, is Professor of Clinical Psychiatry at the Perelman School of Medicine at the University of Pennsylvania. At CHOP, he is Co-Chief, Division of Outpatient Behavioral Health in the Department of Child and Adolescent Psychiatry and Behavioral Sciences, Training Director of the Psychology Internship Program, and a psychologist at the Center for Management of ADHD. In addition to caring for children and families, Dr. Soffer is actively involved in clinical teaching of psychology and psychiatry trainees. He has a long-standing commitment to developing and implementing suicide prevention initiatives, including expanding the use of evidence-based practice in youth suicide risk assessment and intervention in pediatric health care settings.

Preface

This book reflects our many, many years of experience as clinicians and researchers addressing the needs of children with attention-deficit/hyperactivity disorder (ADHD) and supporting their families. We have brought to this task our diverse training backgrounds in school and clinical psychology, our extensive experience in school and pediatric health care settings, and our deep training in school consultation, behavior therapy, family therapy, pediatric school psychology, motivational interviewing, and service delivery with cultural humility. As such, Family–School Success (FSS) is based on several theoretical models and the integration of these frameworks.

The FSS program builds upon empirical research in behavioral parent training and classroom behavioral interventions, which have been shown to be evidence-based treatments for children with ADHD. In addition, FSS highlights the importance of relationships: parent–child, teacher–student, and family–school. In this regard, FSS is unique among behavioral interventions for ADHD in its emphasis on *strengthening relationships while building skills.* This book reflects the strong research base on family involvement in education and our deep belief based on years of experience that interventions for children with ADHD ought to emphasize strengthening the family–school relationship to build teacher–student relationships and promote effective parent–teacher problem solving.

We have been providing FSS to the families of children with ADHD for well over 25 years. The intervention has evolved substantially over time. In the first phase, FSS consisted of a combination of behavioral parent training and behavioral homework intervention and was referred to as *Homework Success* (Power et al., 2001). In the second phase, FSS was expanded to include classroom behavioral interventions, such as the daily report card, and strategies to promote family involvement in education, including family–school collaboration. This adapted version was studied in a randomized controlled trial funded by the National Institute of Mental Health (NIMH; Power et al., 2012). In the third, most recent phase, FSS has been further adapted to emphasize the importance of promoting parental self-discovery and self-empowerment. Incorporating motivational interviewing strategies, FSS now uses a series of well-planned discussions, as opposed to didactic presentations, to help parents understand key concepts and think through how to implement strategies at home and school. As such, we have almost totally rewritten the FSS manual used in our NIMH-funded clinical trial. The manual in this book reflects our most current thoughts about the best way to offer FSS.

The FSS program is a nine-session psychosocial intervention designed for families of children with ADHD who are struggling with impairments in academic, homework, social, emotional, and behavioral functioning. This guidebook provides a comprehensive set of materials for understanding the FSS program, applying the program in practice, examining how it is implemented by practitioners, and evaluating progress.

CHILD AND FAMILY PARTICIPANTS FOR FSS

The FSS program is designed for families of children in grades 1 through 5. The program can be adapted quite readily for use with families of kindergarten and preschool students, but substantive adaptations are likely needed for families of children in grades 6 and above. In Chapter 14 we provide suggestions about how to adapt FSS for the families of younger and older students. Further, we recommend different intervention programs for the families of children who are in grades 6 and above (e.g., Supporting Teens AutoNomy Daily [STAND]; Sibley, 2016). Although the program is intended for families of children with ADHD, it is also appropriate for the broader group of individuals with symptoms and impairment similar to ADHD who may not meet criteria for this disorder. Additionally, FSS was designed for the broad range of children with ADHD, including those with comorbid conditions, such as oppositional defiant disorder, anxiety disorder, mild autism spectrum disorder, and learning disabilities. However, if the primary presenting concerns are impairments due to a comorbid condition as opposed to ADHD, FSS may not be appropriate, and an alternative treatment may be needed. For example, if the primary concern is anxiety preventing a child from going to school, a treatment such as cognitive-behavioral therapy with exposures likely would be indicated. Similarly, if the primary concern is autism spectrum disorder, intensive treatment based upon applied behavior analysis in school and at home likely would be needed.

SERVICE DELIVERY FORMATS FOR FSS

The FSS program was originally designed to be delivered using a combination of in-person group sessions conducted simultaneously with parents and children and family therapy sessions provided individually (Mautone et al., 2012; Power et al., 2012). (Note that we use the term *parents* to refer to individuals who have a legal caregiving role with children or who are authorized by a legal caregiver to serve in this role.) The program has since been adapted as a group intervention for parents only (Morris et al., 2019). In addition, the program has been applied in the context of individualized therapy for children and families with ADHD. This book has been written to support flexibility in implementation, with guidelines for offering sessions using group, individualized, and hybrid formats with children present in sessions and not present. Additionally, the book includes recommendations for implementation of FSS using synchronous telehealth/videoconferencing technology.

COMBINING FSS WITH OTHER INTERVENTIONS

The FSS program can be offered separately or in combination with medication for ADHD. There are clear advantages to offering psychosocial interventions such as FSS separately at the outset of treatment for ADHD, including building critical child and parent skills and strengthening relationships (e.g., parent–child, teacher–student) that are essential for child success in the present and future. In addition, there is evidence that families may become more engaged in psychosocial intervention and thereby derive benefits from this approach if they receive psychosocial intervention prior to medication (Pelham et al., 2016). However, when prior attempts to apply evidence-based psychosocial intervention have not resulted in sufficient improvement and there is a pressing need for symptom reduction, it may be sensible to offer FSS in combination with medication (Barbaresi et al., 2020a).

In general, it is recommended that families receive only one psychosocial intervention at a time. Becoming involved in FSS and another psychosocial intervention simultaneously may not be feasible for families and could detract from family engagement and implementation of strategies for one or both treatments. When children and families require more than one intervention, it is suggested that practitioners collaborate with families to determine the sequence in which they will obtain treatments.

INTENDED READERS OF THIS BOOK

This book is intended for mental health practitioners who work in a range of settings. The book is highly appropriate for school-based mental health practitioners who collaborate with parents and teachers, including school psychologists, school counselors, and school social workers. In fact, the school has many advantages as a venue for FSS service delivery because of its accessibility to families and the opportunities it affords for conjoint family–school collaboration. In addition, services in schools may be publicly funded and offered to families at no financial cost. An issue to consider in offering FSS in schools is that practitioners may need to take additional steps to protect the privacy of information shared, given that schools generally are public places in which information can be shared quite openly.

This book is also very appropriate for clinic-based professionals working in health and mental health organizations, such as pediatric school psychologists, clinical psychologists, clinical social workers, professional counselors, and child and adolescent psychiatrists. Advantages to a clinical setting are that procedures are well established to protect patient privacy and resources may be available to provide additional intervention to families (e.g., pharmacological treatment, other psychosocial intervention) if needed after the program has been completed. Limitations of clinic-based care include operational access barriers (e.g., travel time and expenses, insurance and payment issues) and attitudinal barriers (e.g., perceived stigma about receiving care in a mental health clinic; lack of trust in health systems and providers; Eiraldi et al., 2006).

In addition, this guidebook may be useful for practitioners who provide mental health services in primary care practices. Service delivery in primary care may increase access to services and offer opportunities for integrated psychosocial and medical care (Asarnow et al., 2015). The brief duration of FSS may also be aligned with service delivery models applied in primary care settings, although in some of these practices the typical duration of follow-up care may be briefer than needed to effectively implement FSS (e.g., two to four vs. eight to ten sessions).

This guidebook will be useful for practitioners in practice who wish to expand their skill set for treating families of children with ADHD. Further, it should be helpful for practitioners in training across a range of disciplines (psychology, counseling, social work, child and adolescent psychiatry) as either a text assigned as part of formal coursework or a recommended reading in the context of experiential training (e.g., externship, internship, fellowship).

USE OF THIS BOOK FOR PRACTICE AND RESEARCH

This book is intended primarily for use in schools and clinical practices. The book includes all of the materials needed to deliver FSS, including an explanation of the theoretical and empirical foundation for the program, a detailed manual for implementing each FSS session, specific guidelines for collaborating with teachers, strategies for recruiting participants, handouts for parents, between-session homework assignments for parents, fidelity checklists to examine the quality of intervention implementation, and recommended measures for evaluating intervention outcomes. Chapters 1–4 provide foundational material for implementing the FSS program. The reader is strongly encouraged to read these chapters, and then use the manual described in Chapters 5–13 to implement the program. Chapter 1 provides important background information about the program. Chapter 2 describes the theoretical and empirical justification for the program, Chapter 3 describes how to prepare for delivering FSS, and Chapter 4 presents important information about how to conduct sessions. Chapters 5–13 provide detailed descriptions of the FSS sessions, with handouts and homework assignments organized in Appendix A. The final chapters describe how to adapt FSS for implementation in different contexts and how to evaluate program effectiveness.

The book is intended to address practical issues that arise in delivering FSS to families. The FSS manual in Chapters 5–13 contains numerous "Pro Tips" or practical suggestions for implementing FSS based on our years of experience delivering the program. In addition, in Chapters 3 and 4, we have included a series of vignettes, referred to as "Learning from Our Families," that convey lessons learned through our experience as interventionists. We strongly believe that every family we have served has been a partner with us in considering ways to make the program more helpful and effective.

The book is designed to guide practitioners with the implementation of FSS in its entirety. However, some practitioners may find it useful to extract components of the book to incorporate in the therapy they offer to families of children with ADHD. For example, the sessions on family–school collaboration and behavioral homework intervention as well as strategies for incorporating motivational interviewing could be integrated into another behavioral parent training program being implemented by a practitioner. In addition, providers may find the parent handouts, between-session homework assignments, process fidelity coding system, and some of the progress evaluation measures useful to incorporate into the family therapy work they do.

Although the book is primarily intended for use in practice, it may also be of value to investigators who conduct intervention research with children who have ADHD. The FSS program could be the psychosocial intervention implemented in the context of research evaluating the effectiveness of combining and sequencing psychosocial and pharmacological interventions for children with ADHD (Merrill et al., 2017; Pelham et al., 2016). In addition, the FSS program could be used in the context of intervention research examining the incremental benefits of including children in behavioral parent training; the comparative effectiveness of group versus individualized versus a hybrid of group and individualized care; and the incremental benefit of including an intervention component addressing parental self-regulation (e.g., emotion regulation, organization, time management). Further, the FSS program could be applied in a study investigating the comparative effectiveness of in-person and telehealth approaches to service delivery.

FOUNDATIONAL TRAINING TO IMPLEMENT FSS

FSS is designed to be implemented by licensed and/or certified mental health professionals who are trained to provide intervention to children and their families. It is essential for professionals to have foundational training in behavior therapy. Many excellent books are available to provide instruction in behavior therapy; one that we typically recommend is *Helping the Noncompliant Child* (McMahon & Forehand, 2003). Practitioners also need basic training in school consultation and family–school collaboration; we have found that *Conjoint Behavioral Consultation* (Sheridan & Kratochwill, 2007) provides excellent instruction and guidance in these areas. Effective implementation of FSS requires basic training in motivational interviewing; the text by Miller and Rollnick (2023) is especially useful in providing essential background about this approach to intervention. In addition, effective implementation of FSS requires the ability to work with families in a culturally humble manner; we often recommend the book on cultural humility by Hook and colleagues (2017) to provide guidance in this area.

Acknowledgments

There are so many people who have contributed to this project to whom we are so grateful. We thank Jim Karustis and Dina Habboushe, who were coauthors with Tom Power of another Guilford book, *Homework Success for Children with ADHD*, that served as a foundation for this book. Many components of the Homework Success intervention were incorporated into the Family–School Success (FSS) program, in particular the parts focused on the homework routine and goal-setting tool to support homework performance. In addition, many of the parent handouts included in the *Homework Success* book have been adapted and reprinted in this book. These handouts have proved to be invaluable in our parent training work, and these have been adapted over the years to create the versions that are reprinted in this book.

We are so grateful to our former colleague Jen Betkowski, who provided foundational training to us in motivational interviewing (MI) and assisted us in integrating MI into FSS during the years we had the pleasure to work with her. In addition, we are highly appreciative of the important contributions made by our trainees at Children's Hospital of Philadelphia since the 1990s. Trainees include over 40 fellows, interns, and externs in psychology; fellows in child and adolescent psychiatry; and fellows in developmental and behavioral pediatrics. They have made countless suggestions about how to improve the program curriculum, how to conduct sessions to engage families and promote self-discovery, and how to adapt or create parent handouts. Further, we greatly appreciate the efforts of each member of the research teams involved in the studies we have conducted to develop and evaluate FSS.

We cannot begin to express how grateful we are to the families and teachers who have participated in FSS over the years. We have learned so much from them, and FSS has evolved in large part in response to our experiences working with them and feedback they have shared. It has been an honor for us to serve these families and the teachers of their children.

Finally, we are so grateful to our own families, in particular our spouses and children, who have enabled us to have the careers we have and do the work we enjoy. We thank them for their continual patience and understanding, allowing us to spend time during evenings and weekends to do our work on this book.

Contents

SECTION I. FOUNDATIONS OF THE FAMILY–SCHOOL SUCCESS PROGRAM 1

1. Introduction and Overview 3
    Background Information about Attention-Deficit/Hyperactivity Disorder
        and Evidence-Based Interventions 3
    Major Components of FSS 4
    Theoretical Justification for the Program 5
    Empirical Support for FSS 6
    Unique Features of FSS and This Book 6
        Detailed Manual for Implementing FSS 7
        Handouts for Parents 7
        Between-Session Homework Assignments for Parents 7
        Fidelity Checklists for Promoting High-Quality Implementation 7
        Methods for Assessing Parental Implementation of Intervention Strategies 8
        Measures for Evaluating Child and Family Progress 8
        Strategies for Including Children in FSS 8
        Strategies to Address Parental ADHD 9
        Adapting FSS 9
        Providing FSS with Cultural Humility 10
    How the Book Is Organized 10

2. Theoretical and Empirical Justification for Family–School Success 11
    Theoretical Basis for FSS 12
        Behavioral Psychology 12
        Social Learning Theory 13
        Attachment Theory 13
        Ecological Systems Theory 14
        Self-Determination Theory 14
    Empirical Basis of FSS 15
        Behavioral Parent Training 15
        Behavioral Homework Intervention 16

Conjoint Behavioral Consultation 17
Classroom Behavioral Intervention 17
Motivational Interviewing 18
Coping and Organizational Strategies for Parents 18
Research on FSS 19
Is FSS Acceptable and Feasible? 20
Is FSS Effective? 21
What Predicts Treatment Response? 22
Does Parental Engagement in FSS Make a Difference? 24
How Does FSS Work? 24
Conclusion 25

3. Setting Up the Family–School Success Program 26
Which Children and Families Are Appropriate for FSS? 26
Can FSS Be Implemented Successfully in Schools? 28
Can FSS Be Implemented Successfully in Health and Mental Health Settings? 28
How Can I Recruit Families for FSS? 29
Should I Offer FSS in Groups or Individually? 29
Should Children Be Included in FSS? 30
What Factors Should I Consider in Organizing Groups? 31
Who Can Provide FSS? 31
Can Trainees Have a Role in Providing FSS? 32
Conclusion 32

4. Conducting Family–School Success Sessions 33
How Can I Manage Time Effectively? 34
How Can I Protect Family Privacy and Safety? 34
What Permissions Do I Need to Communicate with Teachers? 35
How Can I Implement FSS to Promote Parent Self-Discovery and Empowerment? 35
How Can I Balance Didactic Presentation and Group Discussion? 36
How Can I Implement FSS with Fidelity and Flexibility? 36
What Strategies Can I Use to Promote Family Engagement? 37
How Can I Work Effectively with Families from Diverse Backgrounds? 38
How Can I Work Effectively with Parents Who Experience Challenges
    during FSS Sessions? 39
What Are Useful Ways to Debrief after Sessions? 39
What Is the Best Way to Use the FSS Manual? 41
Next Steps 42

SECTION II. THE FAMILY–SCHOOL SUCCESS MANUAL 43

5. FSS Session 1: Introduction to the Family–School Success Program 45
Session 1 Agenda 45
Materials Needed 45
Session Process Reminders 46
Goal 1—Welcome families, introductions, and establish relationships among parents and
    program staff. (15 minutes) 46
Goal 2—Introduce program goals, expectations, and "Big Ideas." (20 minutes) 46
Goal 3—Review of ADHD and its relation to behavior and academic performance.
    (15 minutes) 48
Goal 4—Discuss the importance of family involvement in education. (15 minutes) 48

Goal 5—Introduce positive attending strategies. (20 minutes) 49
Goal 6—Assign homework and identify practice supports for consistent implementation. (5 minutes) 50
Session 1 Child Group Agenda 50
Materials Needed 50
Goal 1—Orient children to the components of FSS. 50
Goal 2—Define rules and expectations for the group, and introduce the token reinforcement system. 51
Goal 3—Build group cohesion and relationships. 51
Goal 4—Introduce positive reinforcement. 52
Goal 5—Conclude session. 52

6. FSS Session 2: Strengthening Family Relationships — 53

Session 2 Agenda 53
Materials Needed 53
Session Process Reminders 54
Goal 1—Review homework on positive attending and identify strategies for overcoming barriers to implementation. (25 minutes) 54
Goal 2—Discuss parent coping strategies to promote implementation of effective parenting strategies. (20 minutes) 55
Goal 3—Model Child's Game. (15 minutes) 56
Goal 4—Discuss the key components of Child's Game and provide opportunity for practice with clinician coaching. (25 minutes) 57
Goal 5—Assign homework and identify practice supports for consistent implementation. (5 minutes) 58
Session 2 Child Group Agenda 59
Materials Needed 59
Goal 1—Review the group rules and token reinforcement system. 59
Goal 2—Continue to build group cohesion. 59
Goal 3—Prepare children for Child's Game. 60
Goal 4—Return to parent group to practice Child's Game. 60

7. FSS Session 3: Understanding the Basics of Behavior Management — 61

Session 3 Agenda 61
Materials Needed 61
Session Process Reminders 62
Goal 1—Review homework on practice of Child's Game with a focus on consistent implementation. (20 minutes) 62
Goal 2—Help parents understand and analyze the antecedents and consequences of behavior. (15 minutes) 63
Goal 3—Educate parents about effective ways of giving instructions to their child (antecedent strategy). (10 minutes) 64
Goal 4—Introduce parents to basic consequence strategies for behavior management. (30 minutes) 65
Goal 5—Discuss types of positive reinforcers. (10 minutes) 67
Goal 6—Assign homework and identify practice supports for consistent implementation. (5 minutes) 67
Session 3 Child Group Agenda 68
Materials Needed 68
Goal 1—Review the group rules and token reinforcement system. 68
Goal 2—Maintain group cohesion. 69
Goal 3—Discuss the role of consequences for behavior. 69
Goal 4—Conclude session. 69

8. FSS Session 4: Preparing for Family–School Collaboration   70

Session 4 Agenda   70
Materials Needed   70
Session Process Reminders   71
Goal 1—Review homework assigned last session with a focus on consistent implementation. (20 minutes)   71
Goal 2—Discuss the importance of teacher–student relationship and home–school collaboration. (10 minutes)   72
Goal 3—Discuss ways to build and sustain partnerships with teachers. (25 minutes)   73
Goal 4—Discuss guidelines for establishing a Daily Report Card (DRC). (30 minutes)   75
Goal 5—Assign homework and identify practice supports for consistent implementation. (5 minutes)   76
Session 4 Child Group Agenda   77
Materials Needed   77
Goal 1—Review the group rules and token reinforcement system.   77
Goal 2—Maintain group cohesion.   78
Goal 3—Discuss the importance of the teacher–student relationship.   78
Goal 4—Conclude session.   78

9. FSS Session 5: Introducing the Token Economy   79

Session 5 Agenda   79
Materials Needed   79
Session Process Reminders   80
Goal 1—Review homework assigned last session with a focus on consistent implementation. (25 minutes)   80
Goal 2—Review positive reinforcement and types of reinforcers. (10 minutes)   81
Goal 3—Describe and develop a token economy. (50 minutes)   82
Goal 4—Assign homework and identify practice supports for consistent implementation. (5 minutes)   85
Session 5 Child Group Agenda   85
Materials Needed   85
Goal 1—Review the group rules and token reinforcement system.   85
Goal 2—Maintain group cohesion.   86
Goal 3—Discuss the advantages of a token reinforcement system.   86
Goal 4—Discuss ways to identify reinforcers and promote productive behaviors.   87
Goal 5—Conclude session.   87

10. FSS Session 6: Understanding the Function of Behavior and Establishing the Homework Ritual   88

Session 6 Agenda   88
Materials Needed   88
Session Process Reminders   89
Goal 1—Review homework assigned last session with a focus on consistent implementation. (30 minutes)   89
Goal 2—Assist parents in analyzing the antecedents and consequences of homework behavior. (25 minutes)   90
Goal 3—Support parents in establishing a homework ritual. (30 minutes)   91
Goal 4—Assign homework and identify practice supports for consistent implementation. (5 minutes)   92
Session 6 Child Group Agenda   93
Materials Needed   93
Goal 1—Review the group rules and token reinforcement system.   93

Goal 2—Maintain group cohesion. 94
Goal 3—Discuss homework successes and problems. 94
Goal 4—Help children improve homework routines and identify potential reinforcers. 94
Goal 5—Conclude session. 95

11. FSS Session 7: Managing Time and Goal Setting 96
Session 7 Agenda 96
Materials Needed 96
Session Process Reminders 97
Goal 1—Review homework assigned last session with a focus on consistent implementation. (25 minutes) 97
Goal 2—Assist parents in establishing appropriate time limits for their child to do homework. (20 minutes) 98
Goal 3—Guide parents in helping their children develop time management and goal-setting skills using modeling, role play, and guided practice. (40 minutes) 99
Goal 4—Assign homework and identify practice supports for consistent implementation. (5 minutes) 102
Session 7 Child Group Agenda 102
Materials Needed 102
Goal 1—Review the group rules and token reinforcement system. 103
Goal 2—Maintain group cohesion. 103
Goal 3—Provide children with an overview of the homework goal-setting strategy. 103
Goal 4—Engage children in role-play practice of homework goal setting. 104
Goal 5—Conclude session. 104

12. FSS Session 8: Using Punishment Successfully 105
Session 8 Agenda 105
Materials Needed 105
Session Process Reminders 105
Goal 1—Review homework assigned last session with a focus on consistent implementation. (25 minutes) 106
Goal 2—Provide an overview of the purpose, benefits, and potential adverse effects of punishment. (15 minutes) 107
Goal 3—Discuss strategies for implementing punishment successfully. (45 minutes) 108
Goal 4—Assign homework and identify practice supports for consistent implementation. (5 minutes) 110
Session 8 Child Group Agenda 111
Materials Needed 111
Goal 1—Review the group rules and token reinforcement system. 111
Goal 2—Maintain group cohesion. 112
Goal 3—Discuss experience and progress with homework goal-setting strategies. 112
Goal 4—Discuss appropriate consequences for unproductive and disruptive behavior. 112
Goal 5—Conclude session. 113

13. FSS Session 9: Planning for Future Success 114
Session 9 Agenda 114
Materials Needed 114
Session Process Reminders 115
Goal 1—Review homework assigned at the last session with a focus on consistent implementation. (25 minutes) 115
Goal 2—Support parents in applying FSS strategies to challenging situations. (25 minutes) 116

Goal 3—Guide parents in developing their individual "Formula for Success."
 (30 minutes)   118
Goal 4—Celebrate families' completion of FSS. (10 minutes)   119
Session 9 Child Group Agenda   119
Materials Needed   119
Goal 1—Review the group rules and token reinforcement system.   120
Goal 2—Maintain group cohesion.   120
Goal 3—Discuss the parts of the program children found helpful.   120
Goal 4—Celebrate completion of FSS.   120
Goal 5—Conclude session.   121

SECTION III. ADAPTATIONS AND EVALUATION   123

14. Adaptations across Settings, Populations, and Time of Year   125
How Can I Deliver FSS in Primary Care?   126
How Can I Offer FSS in Private Practice?   126
Can Telehealth Be Used to Deliver FSS?   127
Can I Offer FSS in Individualized Family Sessions?   128
How Do I Modify FSS for Use with Families of Young Children?   129
How Do I Modify FSS for Use with Families of Older Students?   129
What Modifications Are Necessary When Offering FSS in the Summer?   130
What Considerations Should I Keep in Mind When Working with Varying
 Family Constellations?   130
Conclusions   131

15. Assessing Intervention Fidelity, Engagement, and Outcomes   132
with JENELLE NISSLEY-TSIOPINIS

Measures of Intervention Fidelity and Engagement   134
 Content Fidelity   134
 Process Fidelity   134
 Family Engagement   137
 Parental Adherence: Completion of Between-Session Homework Assignments   137
Measures of Family and Family–School Relationship Outcomes   137
Measures of Child Outcomes   138
 Child Functioning at Home: Parent-Report Child Outcome Measures   138
 Child Functioning at School: Teacher-Report Child Outcome Measures   139
Measure of Program Satisfaction   140
Conclusions   140

16. Assessing the Outcomes of Family–School Success   142
with YAEL GROSS and KATIE TREMONT

Context of FSS Program Implementation   143
Program Participants and Intervention Procedures   143
Outcome Measures Administered   144
Results   144
 Program Satisfaction   144
 Intervention Outcomes   145
Conclusions   147

Appendix A. Parent Handouts and Homework Assignments	153
Appendix B. Fidelity Checklists	217
Appendix C. Outcome Measures	229
References	249
Index	255

Purchasers of this book can download and print the reproducible appendices at *www.guilford.com/power2-forms* for personal use or use with students (see copyright page for details).

SECTION I

FOUNDATIONS OF THE FAMILY–SCHOOL SUCCESS PROGRAM

CHAPTER 1

Introduction and Overview

This chapter provides important background information about the Family–School Success (FSS) program, including a description of unique features of the program. More specifically, this chapter describes:

- background information about attention-deficit/hyperactivity disorder (ADHD) and evidence-based interventions
- the major components of FSS
- a brief summary of the theoretical and empirical support for FSS
- unique features of the FSS program and this book

The chapter concludes by describing how the book is organized and how to use the book in practice and research.

BACKGROUND INFORMATION ABOUT ATTENTION-DEFICIT/HYPERACTIVITY DISORDER AND EVIDENCE-BASED INTERVENTIONS

ADHD is a highly common condition; an estimated 10% of children and adolescents are diagnosed with this disorder (Danielson et al., 2018; Visser et al., 2014). ADHD generally results in impairments across multiple domains, including academic and homework performance, family relationships, teacher–student relationships, peer relationships, self-esteem, and behavior compliance (Power et al., 2017). In addition, children with ADHD are at risk for significant impairments in occupational, social, and mental health functioning in adulthood, even if they no longer meet full criteria for this condition by adolescence (Hechtman et al., 2016).

Evidence-based approaches to treating ADHD include psychosocial and pharmacological interventions (Barbaresi et al., 2020a; Wolraich et al., 2019). Although hundreds of studies provide evidence of the efficacy of pharmacological treatment, especially the stimulants, psychosocial interventions provide a critical foundation for intervention by focusing on improving skills (i.e., self-regulation, organization, time management) and strengthening important relationships (e.g., parent–child, teacher–student; DuPaul & Power, 2008; Evans et al., 2019). For the majority of families who view medication as an acceptable treatment for this condition, the combination of psychosocial intervention and medication generally is more effective in reducing ADHD-related impairments than medication alone (Conners et al., 2001; Pelham et al., 2016). For the subset of families who perceive medication as unacceptable, in particular those from groups who historically have been minoritized, psychosocial intervention is the only type of treatment they may receive (Krain et al., 2005), but there are substantial barriers to obtaining this type of treatment in community practice (Weisenmuller & Hilton, 2020).

An important consideration in treating ADHD is that 25–50% of children with this condition have at least one biological parent with ADHD (Takeda et al., 2010). Parents with ADHD generally have more difficulty establishing and maintaining helpful routines for their children, consistently implementing behavioral strategies, and regulating the emotions involved in parenting (Johnston et al., 2012), which may result in poorer outcomes in response to psychosocial intervention (Dawson et al., 2016; Sonuga-Barke et al., 2002). As such, for families in which there is a parent and child with ADHD, it is likely the effects of intervention will be improved by addressing the psychosocial needs of the parent with regard to organization, time management, planning, and emotion regulation (Chronis-Tuscano et al., 2017).

Most psychosocial approaches to intervention for childhood ADHD focus on improving child functioning in either the family or the school (Evans et al., 2018). The intervention described in this book, Family–School Success (FSS), is one of the few approaches that combines evidence-based family and school interventions (see also Pfiffner et al., 2013, 2014). FSS is unique as a family–school intervention in its emphasis on parent–teacher collaboration and problem solving. FSS targets the families of children with ADHD in grades 1–5, although the program can be readily adapted for younger children. The program can be applied with families of children in preschool, although some of the intervention components (i.e., classroom behavioral intervention, behavioral homework intervention) require adaptation for use with younger children. In addition, the program can be applied with families of middle school students, but significant adaptations are required to include a stronger focus on skills training and motivational interviewing for youth (Evans et al., 2016; Sibley et al., 2016).

A distinguishing feature of the FSS program is its major focus on strengthening critical relationships that promote child self-regulation and academic competence (parent–child, family–school, teacher–student). Another hallmark of the program is the emphasis on promoting family self-empowerment to solve problems collaboratively among caregivers and between caregivers and school professionals. FSS was originally designed as a group family intervention that includes children, but it has been adapted so that it can be offered without children present and as an individualized family therapy.

MAJOR COMPONENTS OF FSS

The FSS program includes six main components (see Table 1.1). First, FSS incorporates foundational components of **behavioral parent training,** including modification of behavioral antecedents, positive reinforcement, active ignoring, and strategic punishment (McMahon & Forehand,

TABLE 1.1. Description of the Major Components of FSS

Component of FSS	Example of strategies
Behavioral parent training	Modification of behavioral antecedents (e.g., giving instructions effectively, giving prompts and precorrections) and consequences (e.g., using positive reinforcement for adaptive behaviors frequently; using active ignoring for nonadaptive, high-frequency behaviors; using strategic punishment for targeted behaviors)
Conjoint behavioral consultation	Establishing and strengthening the family–school relationship; collaborating with teachers to develop and sustain a problem-solving partnership to address homework, academic, and behavior concerns
Classroom behavioral intervention	Positively reinforcing teachers for their efforts to apply effective strategies; working with teachers to develop a daily report card (DRC); providing positive reinforcement at home based on DRC ratings
Behavioral homework interventions	Understanding the antecedents of homework behavior; establishing a helpful homework routine; setting reasonable time limits for homework completion; applying goal-setting and time management strategies
Motivational interviewing	Identifying family values and goals; asking open-ended questions; responding to parents with empathy; affirming parents for efforts to change that are consistent with values; rolling with resistance
Coping and organizational strategies for parents	Strengthening parent organization, time management, and planning skills; enhancing parent emotion self-regulation skills; coaching parents to expand their social support network to cope with ADHD and obtain needed services for their child

2003). Second, FSS places emphasis on building a collaborative, problem-solving relationship between parents and teachers, incorporating elements of **conjoint behavioral consultation** (Sheridan & Kratochwill, 2007). Third, FSS includes **classroom behavioral interventions,** in particular the daily report card (DRC), to address concerns at school identified by parents and teachers (DuPaul & Stoner, 2014; Volpe & Fabiano, 2013). Fourth, FSS is distinct in its use of **behavioral homework interventions,** including the implementation of a helpful homework routine and the use of goal-setting and time management strategies (Power et al., 2001). Fifth, FSS sessions are conducted following principles and strategies of **motivational interviewing,** an approach to promote the self-empowerment of individuals to change in a manner that is consistent with their values and goals (Miller & Rollnick, 2023). Sixth, FSS includes a focus on improving **parent coping and organizational skills** in addition to parenting skills, which may enhance the effectiveness of intervention (Chronis-Tuscano et al., 2017). A further description of each component is included in Chapter 2.

THEORETICAL JUSTIFICATION FOR THE PROGRAM

FSS is strongly grounded in several theoretical models related to child development and behavior change. **FSS can be considered a behavioral, social learning, relational, ecological, and**

self-empowering approach to promoting behavior change. First, FSS is rooted in applied behavioral psychology (Patterson, 1982), which highlights that behavioral antecedents and consequences are essential determinants of behavior change. Second, FSS has a strong foundation in social learning theory (Bandura, 1971), affirming that behavior is strongly influenced by observing others, including observations of how behavior is changed by positive reinforcement and punishment. Third, FSS is firmly grounded in attachment theory, which asserts the critical importance of secure, nurturing relationships between children and caregiving adults (e.g., parents, teachers) to promote self-regulation and interpersonal competence (Sroufe et al., 1999). Fourth, FSS is based upon ecological systems theory and strongly emphasizes the critical importance of interactions between systems (i.e., family and school) on child development in each system (Bronfenbrenner, 2009). Finally, FSS is strongly rooted in self-determination theory, emphasizing key factors in promoting the empowerment of caregivers to achieve their goals for parenting (Ryan & Deci, 2018). A more in-depth description of the theoretical underpinnings of FSS is provided in Chapter 2.

EMPIRICAL SUPPORT FOR FSS

Each component of FSS has extensive empirical support. Behavioral parent training and classroom behavior management have been extensively investigated and these approaches are considered well established psychosocial interventions for children with ADHD (Evans et al., 2018; Pelham & Fabiano, 2008). Several randomized controlled studies have demonstrated that conjoint behavioral consultation is an effective approach for promoting family–school collaboration to address targeted academic and behavioral concerns for children, including those with ADHD (Sheridan et al., 2012, 2017). In addition, there is a growing body of literature to support the effectiveness of behavioral homework interventions for children with ADHD (Abikoff et al., 2013; Langberg et al., 2018; Merrill et al., 2017). Further, motivational interviewing has been shown to be an effective approach to changing behavior among children, adolescents, and adults with a wide range of presenting concerns (Miller & Rollnick, 2023), including ADHD (Sibley et al., 2016), and coping and organizational supports can be helpful for parents of children with ADHD (Chronis-Tuscano et al., 2017).

The FSS program in its entirety has also been evaluated by research funded by the National Institute of Mental Health (NIMH) and U.S. Department of Education (MH068290, MH080782). The program has been shown to improve parenting practices, family–school relationships, and child outcomes (Mautone et al., 2012; Power et al., 2012). Empirical support for the multicomponent FSS program as well as its components is described in detail in Chapter 2.

UNIQUE FEATURES OF FSS AND THIS BOOK

This book is designed as a guidebook for practitioners who work with children with ADHD and their families in settings such as clinical practices, schools, and primary care. The following are some of the unique features of this book.

Detailed Manual for Implementing FSS

The book includes a detailed, session-by-session manual for how to implement the FSS program. The manual emphasizes for practitioners the importance of building on the insights and experience of each parent and the collective wisdom of the group. Unlike most behavioral parent training programs, didactic presentations of parenting strategies are designed to be very brief. In contrast, education in FSS is generally provided through group discussion, and parents are guided through a process of self-discovery. A hallmark of the manual is a series of open-ended questions to guide discussions in a manner that builds on parents' current knowledge and skills, offers opportunities for parents to support each other in exploring alternative actions, and provides affirmation to parents for efforts to change and implement new strategies.

Handouts for Parents

Included in Appendix A are handouts for parents to promote their understanding of behavior-change approaches and guide them in implementing recommended strategies. The handouts are designed to complement information discussed in each FSS session and in some ways take the place of didactic presentations of the material during sessions. Each session of FSS includes at least one parent handout.

Between-Session Homework Assignments for Parents

Our research on FSS has demonstrated that parental completion of homework assignments between sessions is associated with better outcomes with regard to parenting practices and child behavior change (Clarke et al., 2015; Morris et al., 2019). Parents are given at least one homework assignment after each program session. The homework assignment is designed to encourage them to implement and practice strategies that were discussed during the session. At the end of each homework assignment, parents are asked to identify any challenges they encountered in implementing the strategy and potential solutions to support them in working through difficulties with implementation. These homework assignments are used to guide discussion during FSS sessions focused on the rationale for each strategy and suggestions to support consistent implementation of recommendations. A full set of between-session homework assignments are included in Appendix A of this book.

Fidelity Checklists for Promoting High-Quality Implementation

The book includes checklists to promote high-quality implementation of FSS sessions and to evaluate the degree to which components of each session have been implemented as intended (see Appendix B). A set of content fidelity checklists is included to determine whether the steps and components of the session have been implemented by clinicians. In addition, a process fidelity checklist is included to examine the extent to which clinicians have implemented motivational interviewing and group process strategies (e.g., promoting change talk, facilitating connections among parents, maintaining the focus of participants on evidence-based strategies).

Methods for Assessing Parental Implementation of Intervention Strategies

Research has shown that parental implementation of strategies learned in behavioral parent training programs is associated with a favorable response to intervention (Clarke et al., 2015; Morris et al., 2019; Rooney et al., 2018). We recommend two strategies for examining intervention implementation. One method is to collect and score homework the session after it is assigned to parents; these assignments can readily be scored for degree of completion (Clarke et al., 2015). The codebook for scoring between-session homework assignments is included in Appendix C. Another method is for clinicians to use a Likert scale to rate parental implementation of each homework assignment based upon parental reports during the homework review period at the beginning of each session (Rooney et al., 2018).

Measures for Evaluating Child and Family Progress

The book includes several measures assessing variables targeted by the FSS program, including scales assessing child behavior, parenting practices, and the family–school relationship. A major consideration in identifying measures for assessing child and family progress has been to select scales that are relatively brief and feasible to use in practice as well as research. For the assessment of changes in child behavior, we have included a parent-report measure assessing child ADHD, externalizing symptoms, and internalizing symptoms, as well as child strengths (e.g., self-regulation, and interpersonal competence; Mautone et al., 2020; Power, Koshy, et al., 2013). To assess reductions in impairment, we recommend a parent- and teacher-report measure commonly used in assessing the broad range of impairments associated with ADHD (Fabiano et al., 2006). In addition, because FSS has such a strong focus on improving student homework behavior, we have included a parent- and teacher-report measure of homework performance (Power et al., 2015).

The FSS program is effective in part because it changes parenting practices, specifically by reducing negative and ineffective parenting practices (Booster et al., 2016). As such, we have included a parent-report measure of negative/ineffective parenting (Furman & Giberson, 1995). Further, a major target of change for the FSS program is the family–school relationship, so we have included a parent- and teacher-report measure of this variable (Kohl et al., 2000).

Strategies for Including Children in FSS

The FSS program was originally designed to include children in most of the sessions. In fact, the version of FSS evaluated by a NIMH-funded randomized controlled trial included children in the intervention (Power et al., 2012). For many of the sessions, parents and children met in separate groups simultaneously and came together at designated times. The purpose of including children is to prepare them to work on strategies their parents are learning and to offer parents and children opportunities to learn and practice skills together in session. As a rule, we recommend the inclusion of children in the program, but we understand that it is sometimes not feasible to do so because of the additional staff needed to conduct separate parent and child group meetings and the preparation time involved. For clinicians who are able to involve children in sessions, the book includes detailed guidelines for conducting sessions with children present.

Strategies to Address Parental ADHD

Because so many parents of children with ADHD have symptoms of this condition themselves (Chronis-Tuscano et al., 2017), the FSS program incorporates strategies to assist parents in managing the aspects of ADHD that can have an effect on parenting. The program includes an explicit focus on helping parents identify challenges they encounter in implementing behavioral interventions and develop strategies to address these. A major portion of Session 2 is devoted to helping parents understand how their own attention, organization, and self-control difficulties can have an effect on their parenting practices. This session includes a discussion of strategies to enable parents to be better organized in implementing family routines, more successful in regulating their emotional reactions to their children's misbehavior (e.g., frustration, hurt, anger), and more effective in seeking out and obtaining needed support from other caregivers, relatives, and friends.

Adapting FSS

The FSS program was originally designed to be offered in groups with students in grades 1–5. However, the program can be adapted quite readily for individualized care, with younger children, and in a range of settings. This section briefly describes these adaptations. For further discussion see Chapter 14.

There are clear advantages to involving parents in groups, such as offering parents opportunities to learn from and support each other. However, a noteworthy limitation of group care is that sessions are conducted on a fixed schedule, which may serve as a barrier for some families. In contrast, individualized care may offer more flexibility in scheduling and provides ongoing opportunities to tailor strategies to the individual needs of each family. In addition, it is much more practical to involve children when FSS is provided on an individualized basis to families.

Adaptations of the program are needed for kindergarten and preschool students who usually are not assigned homework by teachers. Young children are involved in educational activities in the home and the strategies in FSS can be adapted to support children in performing these tasks.

The FSS program can be applied in schools, clinics based in health and mental health organizations, primary care practices, and private practices. There are tremendous advantages to providing the program in schools, in particular the enhanced opportunities for practitioners to become involved in conjoint family–school collaboration and the increased feasibility of collecting progress evaluation data from teachers. Health and mental health settings are appropriate for delivering FSS, and families often seek out services for ADHD in these venues. In addition, primary care practices that include integrated or co-located behavioral health clinicians may be well suited as a venue for service delivery and may reduce some barriers to care, including reduced stigma associated with accessing behavioral health care. The FSS program and similar parent training programs are often provided using telehealth methods (Fogler et al., 2020), which may also reduce barriers to accessing the program. See Chapter 14 for details.

Providing FSS with Cultural Humility

The FSS program has evolved substantially over the years to be responsive to families from diverse backgrounds. The infusion of motivational interviewing strategies into every session of the program has been highly useful in enabling clinicians to practice with cultural humility. In particular, practitioners are trained to ask open-ended questions, listen carefully, reflect empathy, identify family values and goals, roll with resistance, and affirm family efforts to change in the direction consistent with family values and goals. In addition, the training of practitioners involves ongoing inquiry into the dynamics of privilege and oppression to identify potential ways that systemic and structural factors (e.g., barriers to access and engagement), clinician identity (e.g., age, race, ethnicity, cultural background, religion, gender identity, and sexual orientation), parent identity, and perceptions of the other's identity may contribute to the marginalization of families (Nixon, 2019).

HOW THE BOOK IS ORGANIZED

This book is organized into three sections (see Table 1.2). Section I (Chapters 1–4) provides a foundation for the FSS program. It summarizes the theoretical and empirical support for the program, and it describes how to set up the program and conduct sessions. Section II (Chapters 5–13) contains the program manual, that is, a detailed description of how to conduct each session. Each chapter in this section is focused on describing how to implement the nine core sessions of FSS. Section III (Chapters 14–16) describes how to adapt the program across settings and how to evaluate intervention fidelity and progress. The book also includes several appendices, which provide clinicians with useful resources for conducting and evaluating FSS. Included in the appendices are parent handouts and between-session homework assignments for parents, intervention fidelity checklists, and measures for assessing child and family progress and program satisfaction.

TABLE 1.2. How This Book Is Organized

Sections of the book	Chapters
I. Foundations of the Family–School Success Program	Chapter 1. Introduction and Overview Chapter 2. Theoretical and Empirical Justification for Family–School Success Chapter 3. Setting Up the Family–School Success Program Chapter 4. Conducting Family–School Success Sessions
II. The Family–School Success Manual	Chapters 5–13. Program Manual for Nine Family–School Success Sessions
III. Adaptations and Evaluation	Chapter 14. Adaptations across Settings, Populations, and Time of Year Chapter 15. Assessing Intervention Fidelity, Engagement, and Outcomes Chapter 16. Assessing the Outcomes of Family–School Success

CHAPTER 2

Theoretical and Empirical Justification for Family–School Success

Evidence-based interventions for ADHD include pharmacological and psychosocial approaches (Barbaresi et al., 2020a; Wolraich et al., 2019). Research and guidelines from professional organizations have affirmed that psychosocial interventions are an important foundation for treatment due to their focus on skill building. For example, behavioral parent training, which typically includes group or individual family sessions focused on increasing the use of positive parenting strategies and reducing ineffective discipline strategies, has been shown to improve family relationships, parenting practices, and child functioning at home (Evans et al., 2018; McMahon & Forehand, 2003). In addition, classroom behavioral interventions, such as contingency management and the DRC, are effective strategies to improve child behavior at school (Evans et al., 2018; Volpe & Fabiano, 2013). Skills training focused on organization, time management, and planning skills can be helpful to improve children's ability to complete tasks such as homework and chores (Abikoff et al., 2013; Evans et al., 2011; Langberg et al., 2012).

As noted in Chapter 1, FSS is an evidence-based, multicomponent psychosocial intervention. This chapter provides a more in-depth description of the theoretical and empirical foundation for FSS than was included in Chapter 1 and describes the strength of the evidence for the program. This chapter will help the reader understand why FSS includes certain components and why it is delivered using motivational interviewing strategies. In addition, the chapter provides evidence for why FSS is likely to be successful in strengthening the family–school relationship and improving parenting and child outcomes. The following topics are addressed in this chapter:

- Theoretical basis for FSS
- Empirical basis for interventions similar to FSS
  - Goals of FSS
  - Components of FSS

- Research evaluating the FSS program
  - Is FSS acceptable and feasible?
  - Is FSS effective?
  - What factors predict response to FSS?
  - Does parent engagement in FSS make a difference?
  - How does FSS work?

THEORETICAL BASIS FOR FSS

FSS focuses on fostering parent use of effective behavior-change strategies in the context of collaborative and supportive relationships to address child ADHD. In other words, parents learn to teach and model appropriate behavior and to work effectively with other important adults in children's lives (e.g., teachers, other caregivers) to support generalization into settings outside the home. The program is grounded in behavioral, social learning, attachment, ecological systems, and self-determination theories. The following sections provide an overview of the theoretical foundation for FSS.

Behavioral Psychology

According to behavioral theory, behavior is shaped by the environment. Specifically, the environmental conditions prior to the performance of the behavior, or antecedents, set the stage for the child's behavior. Events that occur immediately after the performance of the behavior, or consequences, influence whether the behavior is likely to continue in the future. The strategic adjustment of consequences on behavior change is known as operant conditioning (Skinner, 1976). The premise is that environmental events, both antecedents and consequences, can be altered to promote behavior change (Kazdin, 2005).

A key component of behavioral theory is a focus on observable, measurable behaviors as targets of behavior change. In other words, when identifying a goal for behavior change, that goal should be something specific that everyone can see or hear. For example, telling a child that the goal is "listening" is somewhat vague and potentially hard to evaluate. Instead, the goal could be "following directions the first time." In this case, we would be able to observe the child engaging in an action consistent with the direction that was given, indicating compliance with the expectation.

Behavior that is reinforced, or rewarded, will likely continue or increase in frequency. Positive reinforcement occurs when a desired item or experience is offered in response to a behavior. For example, a child might be given a new toy or the opportunity to stay up late as a result of meeting a behavioral expectation. Negative reinforcement is when an undesired item or situation is removed when an expectation is met. For example, a child might earn a brief break from homework as reinforcement for working productively for an identified period.

There are two primary ways to reduce the occurrence of a behavior—ignoring and punishment. Ignoring is the purposeful act of not providing reinforcement (or punishment) in response to a behavior. Behaviors that are ignored temporarily increase in frequency before decreasing; this increase is referred to as an extinction burst. Two types of punishment can be used to reduce the occurrence of undesired behavior: positive and negative punishment. In situations involving positive punishment, an aversive consequence is applied after the performance of an undesired behavior. For example, if a child engages in physical aggression with a sibling, a parent might provide corrective feedback to the child. Negative punishment, on the other hand, involves removal of something desirable as a consequence for the undesired behavior. In this case, the child who fought with the sibling might lose access to a favorite toy for a period of time as a result of the aggressive behavior.

Social Learning Theory

Social learning theory expands on behavioral theory to recognize the influence that observing others has on behavior. The influence of reinforcement and punishment on behavior through operant conditioning is acknowledged as one important component of learning. Additionally, according to social learning theory, behavior is influenced by observing, modeling, and imitating others (Bandura, 1971). Behavior can be learned virtually automatically through observation of the consequences experienced by others; direct instruction or practice is not necessarily required.

It is important to consider the mediational cognitive processes that influence the acquisition of behavior. Attention to the person serving as a model, retention (i.e., ability to remember what was observed), reproduction (i.e., ability to perform the observed behavior), and motivation or desire to perform or not perform the behavior all play a role in learning (Bandura, 1977). Learning will happen most easily when developmentally appropriate tasks are presented clearly and in a motivating way.

Finally, according to social learning theory, just as individual behavior is influenced by the environment, the environment is influenced by individual behavior. This concept is called reciprocal determinism (Bandura, 1977). For example, if a child repeatedly struggles to follow directions until a parent removes a privilege, the parent learns that punishment is necessary to elicit a response from the child, and the child learns that a response is not required until the parent issues a punishment.

Attachment Theory

Attachment theory emphasizes the central importance of secure, supportive relationships for healthy development (Sroufe et al., 2005). Development and adaptation depend upon early childhood relationships, in particular the parent–child attachment, as well as the quality of ongoing relationships. Insecure attachments related to harsh and/or inconsistent parenting early in life can initiate a pathway leading to child and adolescent psychopathology. However, subsequent relational experiences during childhood and adolescence, such as warm and emotionally supportive parent–child relationships, can decrease risk and initiate health-promoting pathways (Sroufe, 2016).

Secure, affirming parent–child relationships during childhood promote child self-regulation and interpersonal competence not only in the family context but also in systems outside the home, including school (Pianta, 1999). In other words, strengthening the parent–child relationship has the potential to set the child up for school success by preparing the child to engage in rule-governed behavior in school and enabling the child to establish and maintain positive relationships with teachers and peers.

Attachment theory has been extended to highlight the critical importance of the teacher–student relationship. Supportive, nonconflictual teacher–student relationships further support the development of child self-regulation skills and interpersonal competence, which can result in greater academic engagement, improvements in academic achievement, and success in relating with peers (Hamre et al., 2008).

Ecological Systems Theory

Ecological systems theory extends influences on child development beyond individual relationships to include the impact of multiple levels of the child's environment (Bronfenbrenner, 2009). Specifically, according to this theory, child development is conceptualized as occurring within a set of nested contexts (e.g., family, school, larger community, political system), each of which has an influence on the others. The individuals in the child's immediate environment (e.g., parents, teachers, peers, siblings) and interactions between these individuals (e.g., parent–teacher relationships) are considered the most influential in fostering child development. That said, other contexts that do not include the child directly often do have substantial impact on child development. For example, if a parent or caregiver experiences substantial stress at work, their heightened stress level can have a negative impact on parent–child interactions. Finally, ecological systems theory acknowledges that even broader contextual influences, such as sociopolitical climate, influence caregiving practices and have an impact on child development.

According to ecological systems theory, development occurs as a result of dynamic, bidirectional processes between systems in addition to within systems. For example, child academic progress is influenced by interactions between the child and teachers as well as the connection (or lack of a connection) between the family and the school. Similarly, behavior change for a child with ADHD or other chronic condition may be influenced by interactions within the family, school, and health system as well as connections among these systems of care (Power & Bradley-Klug, 2013).

Self-Determination Theory

Self-determination theory (SDT) is a framework for understanding motivation, including how and why people change (Deci & Ryan, 1985; Ryan & Deci, 2018). SDT differentiates autonomous motivation (i.e., intrinsic motivation and extrinsic motivation that has been integrated into one's personal values) from controlled motivation (i.e., motivation regulated by external sources, including approval from others and avoidance of shame). Autonomous motivation is associated with greater initiation and sustainment of health-promoting behaviors and better health outcomes than controlled motivation.

According to SDT, an individual's level of autonomous motivation in pursuing goals is associated with the fulfillment of three sets of needs. First, motivation is stronger when individuals believe they can determine goals for themselves and make decisions leading to the achievement of goals. Second, motivation is associated with a belief that one has the skills, or is capable of acquiring the skills, needed to attain important goals. Third, motivation is strongly influenced by a person's connectedness with others and the degree to which a person feels supported in working toward identified goals. SDT is closely associated with motivational interviewing (MI) and offers a theoretical model for understanding how MI can promote meaningful and sustained change in the context of intervention (Ryan & Deci, 2008).

EMPIRICAL BASIS OF FSS

The FSS program has been designed to accomplish three major goals: (1) strengthen parenting practices and the parent–child relationship, (2) improve family involvement in education and family–school collaboration, and (3) strengthen parent effectiveness in supporting the child at home and school. FSS has multiple components to achieve these goals, including behavioral parent training (McMahon & Forehand, 2003) and behavioral homework intervention (Power et al., 2001), conjoint behavioral consultation (Sheridan & Kratochwill, 2007), classroom behavioral intervention, such as the DRC (Volpe & Fabiano, 2013), motivational interviewing (Miller & Rollnick, 2023), and strategies to support parental coping and organization. See Figure 2.1 for an illustration of the goals of FSS and how FSS is proposed to have an effect on child functioning at home and school. See Table 2.1 for a description of the FSS components that address each goal. Each component is described in more detail below.

Behavioral Parent Training

As noted above, behavioral parent training (BPT) is a well-established treatment for children with ADHD and has been shown to have a positive impact on child- and family-centered outcomes, including child functioning at home, parenting practices, and family relationships

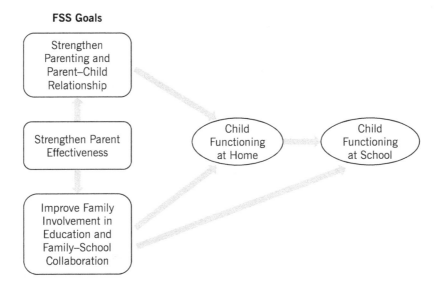

FIGURE 2.1. Theory of change for FSS. FSS is designed to accomplish three goals: (1) strengthen parenting skills and the parent–child relationship, (2) improve family involvement in education and family–school collaborative relationships, and (3) strengthen parental effectiveness in supporting the child at home and school. Addressing these goals can improve child functioning at home as well as in school.

TABLE 2.1. Components of FSS Associated with Each Program Goal

FSS goal	Associated FSS components
Strengthen parenting and parent–child relationship	• Behavioral parent training
Improve family involvement in education and family–school collaboration	• Behavioral homework intervention • Conjoint behavioral consultation • Classroom behavioral interventions, including daily report card
Strengthen parent effectiveness to support children at home and school	• Motivational interviewing • Strategies to support parental coping and organization

(Evans et al., 2018; McMahon & Forehand, 2003). BPT programs typically include 6 to 16 group or individual family therapy sessions and focus on teaching parents how to use positive parenting strategies to change the contingencies at home to increase the likelihood that children will display appropriate or desired behavior (Pelham & Fabiano, 2008). Decades of research related to BPT have illustrated the effectiveness of this approach for addressing child ADHD (Evans et al., 2018; Pelham & Fabiano, 2008; Pelham et al., 1998).

Early evaluations of BPT often focused on comparisons between a specific BPT program and a comparison condition to evaluate whether BPT resulted in improvements in ADHD symptoms, impairment, and parenting skills (e.g., MTA Cooperative Group, 1999; Sonuga-Barke et al., 2001). More recent research has focused on understanding what works best for specific populations (e.g., single parents, parents with ADHD or depression, families with financial need; Evans et al., 2018).

Although behavioral parent training is considered a well-established treatment that results in reduced impairment at home, this intervention generally is not as effective in improving performance in other environments (e.g., school; Evans et al., 2018). It is not surprising that strategies focused on the home setting are less effective in changing behavior in other environments with different demands and structure. This is an important component in the justification for including in FSS an explicit focus on the development of collaborative family–school partnerships and on interventions that are likely to result in reduced educational impairment.

Behavioral Homework Intervention

Homework is an important target of intervention for children and youth with ADHD. Homework performance in elementary school has been shown to be associated with academic achievement in high school (Langberg et al., 2011). In addition, homework problems can be the source of conflictual parent–child interactions and family–school relationships, which can contribute to child impairment in the home and school settings (Power et al., 2001).

Since 2010, numerous interventions targeting students in elementary, middle, and high school have been shown to improve the organizational skills and homework performance of students with ADHD (Bikic et al., 2017). These interventions differ in the extent to which they use a parent training versus a child skills training approach. Parent training approaches typically focus on changes in behavioral antecedents (e.g., homework routine, goal-setting and time management strategies) and consequences (e.g., positive reinforcement using token systems) to improve homework performance. They may also integrate classroom behavioral interventions (e.g., DRC) targeting behaviors related to homework organization and completion (Merrill et al., 2016). Child skills training approaches generally focus on improving homework tracking, materials management, time management, and planning skills (Abikoff et al., 2013; Evans et al., 2014; Langberg et al., 2018; Pfiffner et al., 2018), although these approaches differ with regard to the extent to which they focus on learning and mastering skills (e.g., Abikoff et al., 2013) versus executing skills on a consistent basis (e.g., Langberg et al., 2018). Evidence-based skills training approaches for improving organizational skills and homework performance typically include a parent training component to promote generalization and sustainment of intervention effects.

Parent training approaches appear more effective with young elementary-age students, but there is evidence that parenting training and child skills approaches may be equally effective by the later elementary years (Abikoff et al., 2013). In addition, skills training approaches likely are more effective at the middle school and high school levels.

Conjoint Behavioral Consultation

Family involvement in education, including collaboration between families and schools, has positive impacts on children's engagement in school, attitudes toward school, and academic performance (Anderson & Minke, 2007; Christenson & Sheridan, 2001; Epstein, 1995). The conjoint behavioral consultation (CBC) model (Sheridan & Kratochwill, 2007) is an effective model for promoting strong, collaborative partnerships between families and schools. The model includes four steps: (1) conjoint problem identification, (2) conjoint problem analysis, (3) intervention implementation, and (4) conjoint intervention evaluation. Throughout the process, parents and teachers work together closely, with the support of a consultant, to develop and implement strategies to support student behavior and performance.

Numerous research studies have illustrated that CBC is an effective model for addressing children's academic, behavioral, and social difficulties (Sheridan et al., 2014), including for children with ADHD (Gormley et al., 2020; Sheridan et al., 2012, 2017). Specifically, studies have shown that when parents and teachers work together using the CBC model, children's off-task behavior decreases and on-task behavior and social interactions improve based on teacher-report and direct observation of student behavior in the classroom (Sheridan et al., 2017). Additionally, the use of the CBC model results in more positive, collaborative relationships between parents and teachers, and this relationship mediates the effect of CBC on student outcomes (Sheridan et al., 2012, 2017). In other words, when parents and teachers work together effectively and develop collaborative relationships, students have more positive educational and behavioral outcomes.

Classroom Behavioral Intervention

Classroom behavioral intervention, also known as behavioral contingency management in the classroom, has been considered a well-established treatment for ADHD for many years (Pelham et al., 1998; Pelham & Fabiano, 2008). Numerous studies illustrate that teacher use of contingency management strategies (e.g., rewards, token economies, time out) results in reductions in ADHD symptoms and improvements in targeted areas of impairment (e.g., social skills, on-task behavior in the classroom, work completion; Chronis et al., 2004; Fabiano et al., 2007).

Research has also focused on the use of the DRC intervention to combine classroom behavioral intervention with opportunities for rewards at home contingent on appropriate classroom behavior (Volpe & Fabiano, 2013). DRCs also provide an opportunity for parents and teachers to communicate consistently about child performance in the classroom. Typically, the DRC is developed with support of a consultant. Goals might include behavioral targets (e.g., on-task behavior, raising a hand when the student wants to speak) or academic goals (e.g., work accuracy, work completion). When CBC approaches are used, parents and teachers collaborate to develop mutually identified goals, which can be incorporated into a DRC. Studies have illustrated that the DRC intervention results in improvements in classroom behavior and academic productivity (e.g., Fabiano et al., 2010; Owens et al., 2012).

Motivational Interviewing

Unlike the components of FSS described above that focus on what is delivered during intervention (i.e., content of intervention), motivational interviewing (MI) emphasizes how intervention is delivered (i.e., process of intervention). MI is an approach to intervention that promotes client motivation to change and investment in implementing change strategies (Miller & Rollnick, 2023). This approach is inherently collaborative in nature; the focus is on building a partnership with families that creates a safe, supportive context for exploration, self-reflection, and risk taking. In contrast to didactic approaches that emphasize imparting knowledge to others, MI affirms the wisdom of participants and seeks to elicit insights from them that can lead to new ways of behaving.

MI has several fundamental principles (Miller & Rollnick, 2023). First, it is critical for the therapist to *listen with empathy,* which builds trust, conveys acceptance of participant ambivalence about change, and encourages active exploration. Second, the role of the therapist is to examine ambivalence and *clarify the discrepancy* between how a person aspires to behave (i.e., critical values and goals for self and family) and how one is actually behaving (i.e., current actions). Third, when participants show evidence of opposing change, it is important for the therapist to *roll with resistance,* avoid direct conflict, look for examples when participants are essentially arguing with themselves, and then highlight the discrepancy (i.e., internal conflict within the participant). Fourth, the role of the therapist is to *support self-efficacy* (i.e., a belief that one is able to achieve identified goals) by affirming behaviors suggesting a willingness to change, including questioning one's current beliefs and actions, taking the risk to try a new way of behaving, and soliciting feedback from others.

Coping and Organizational Strategies for Parents

The parents of children with ADHD often have coping difficulties that contribute to challenges with parenting. Approximately 25–50% of families in which there is a child with ADHD have at least one biological parent with this condition (Takeda et al., 2010), and many of these individuals have comorbid mental health conditions. Elevated symptoms of ADHD may pose unique challenges to parents in the areas of cognitive processing (e.g., organization, planning, working memory) and self-regulation of behavior and emotions (Johnston et al., 2012), which can have an impact on their parenting. In addition, there is evidence that behavioral interventions may be less effective in improving child outcomes in families in which there is a parent with ADHD (Chronis-Tuscano et al., 2017) and that the presence of parental ADHD may mitigate the maintenance of gains from behavioral intervention (Dawson et al., 2016).

To address parent coping challenges, interventions for families of children with ADHD have been adapted to include components to address parental mental health difficulties including symptoms of ADHD and depression (Chronis-Tuscano et al., 2017). These components may include cognitive behavioral and executive-functioning training approaches designed to target cognitive processes and self-regulation functions implicated in ADHD. These approaches often target organization, time management, planning, self-control of behavior, and the management of stress and emotions.

RESEARCH ON FSS

FSS was originally developed and evaluated with funding from NIMH and the U.S. Department of Education in two different projects. The primary project was a large-scale clinical trial focused on children with ADHD in grades 2–6 (Power et al., 2012). The primary goal of the study was to evaluate whether FSS was more effective than the control group in improving parenting practices, the quality of the family–school relationship, child academic performance, including homework performance, and reducing ADHD and oppositional defiant symptoms at home and school. The second project was a smaller pilot study designed to develop and evaluate an adaptation of FSS for young children with ADHD in kindergarten and first grade (Mautone et al., 2012). The purpose of this pilot was to determine whether the modified version of FSS was acceptable to participants, was feasible to implement, and resulted in improvements in parenting practices, family involvement in education, and child functioning at home and school.

For the large-scale clinical trial, our team enrolled 199 children in grades 2–6 with ADHD Combined or Inattentive presentations according to parent report on the Schedule for Affective Disorders and Schizophrenia for School-Age Children—*DSM-IV* (K-SADS-P IVR; Ambrosini, 2000). Enrolled children also had elevated (> 85th percentile) symptoms of inattention and/or hyperactivity on teacher rating scales and evidence of educational impairment (i.e., score at or above 0.75 standard deviations above the mean on the Homework Problem Checklist; Anesko et al., 1987). Children with autism, intellectual disabilities, and severe internalizing disorders were excluded. Children on medication were included. Families were offered a medication trial as part of the study. If the family elected to have the child take medication to treat ADHD during the study, medication type and dose were titrated and stabilized prior to enrollment in the psychosocial interventions.

Once families were enrolled, they were randomized to receive either FSS or a comparison condition known as Coping with ADHD through Relationships and Education (CARE); interventions were delivered in an outpatient behavioral health clinic with a specialty ADHD program. The version of FSS used in the clinical trial included 12 weekly sessions: 6 multifamily group sessions with concurrent parent and child groups, 4 individualized family sessions, and 2 conjoint family–school consultation sessions held at the child's school. In addition, clinicians contacted the child's teacher by phone twice during the intervention to monitor progress and refine interventions as needed. The first session was 3 hours; all remaining group sessions were 90 minutes; individual family sessions were 60 minutes; and school consultations were approximately 45 minutes. Families received homework assignments at each session designed to support parent skills practice and implementation. In the clinical trial, an average of 7 (range 3–10) families participated in each FSS cohort.

CARE is an active control condition designed to control for the nonspecific effects of intervention. CARE does not include any of the primary components of FSS or training in the use of evidence-based interventions for ADHD. Instead, the goal is to provide support and education to families of children with ADHD. Specifically, sessions include discussion of child progress at home and school, generic education about ADHD, and a focus on encouraging parents to support each other in coping with their children's difficulties. The version of CARE used in the clinical trial included 11 group sessions (concurrent parent and child groups) and one school meeting.

Outcomes included intervention acceptability, family involvement in education, the quality of the parent–child and parent–teacher relationships, child homework and academic performance reported by parents and teachers, and ADHD and oppositional defiant symptoms as reported by parents and teachers. For additional information about the clinical trial, see Power et al. (2012). Many of the measures used in the clinical trial are useful to monitor progress and evaluate outcomes when FSS is implemented in practice.

As noted above, the pilot study focused on younger children with ADHD was designed to adapt FSS for implementation with families of kindergarten and first-grade students with ADHD (Mautone et al., 2012). The modified version of FSS, known as FSS—Early Elementary (FSS-EE) was developed through an iterative process over a 6-month period, based on a review of the literature, consultation with experts, focus groups with parents and teachers of young children with ADHD, and an initial trial of the program with a small group of families. The study included an examination of intervention acceptability, family involvement in education, parenting practices, and child functioning at home and school. For additional details, see Mautone et al. (2012); see Chapter 15 and Appendix B for suggested progress monitoring/outcome evaluation procedures and sample measures.

Is FSS Acceptable and Feasible?

Our research indicates that FSS is acceptable to caregivers, children, and school staff, and it is feasible to implement. To evaluate acceptability in all of our studies, we obtained parent, child, and teacher ratings on psychometrically sound measures of treatment acceptability. In the large-scale clinical trial (Power et al., 2012), parent ratings of the acceptability of FSS were high and significantly higher than scores for CARE (active control condition). Teachers and children also provided ratings indicating high levels of acceptability for FSS, although their ratings were not significantly different than those of teachers and children in the CARE group. In the pilot study with families of children in kindergarten and first grade, parents and teachers again indicated high ratings of program acceptability for FSS-EE (Mautone et al., 2012). Similar to the large-scale study, parent ratings of acceptability of FSS-EE were significantly higher than those for CARE.

FSS and FSS-EE are both feasible for clinicians to implement and for parents to attend regularly. In the large trial, seven different clinicians delivered the FSS intervention to the 100 enrolled families. Eighty-eight teachers also participated in the family–school consultation components of the intervention. FSS group leaders delivered the intervention with a high degree of fidelity to the manual, and families had high rates of session attendance. Over 90% of families attended at least 9 of the 12 sessions. Adherence to between-session homework assignments was variable, which suggests that clinicians might want to incorporate strategies to support successful intervention implementation at home and school. In the pilot trial for FSS-EE, groups were administered by three different clinicians to 29 families; 24 teachers participated in the family–school consultation sessions. Rates of content fidelity, attendance, and adherence to homework were similar to those in the larger trial.

Our team has continued to monitor acceptability and feasibility for an adapted version of FSS that we implement in the context of an outpatient specialty ADHD program. Parent ratings indicate that families consider the clinic-based version of FSS to be very helpful (Morris et al., 2019). Also, attendance at sessions suggests that the program is feasible for parents to attend and for clinicians to administer. Completion of between-session homework assignments continued to be somewhat variable, highlighting that some families may need additional support to practice at home.

Is FSS Effective?

Consistent with findings from many other evaluations of behavioral interventions for children with ADHD (e.g., Evans et al., 2018), our research illustrates that participation in FSS has a positive impact on parenting practices and child functioning at home and school. Like other studies (e.g., Langberg et al., 2010; Wells et al., 2000), our work demonstrated significant reductions in child inattention/avoidance during homework and parent use of negative and ineffective discipline strategies. Reductions in parent use of negative and ineffective discipline were maintained through the 3-month follow-up period.

Our research also extended previous studies in important ways. First, our work has shown that FSS can improve the quality of the parent–teacher relationship, parent self-efficacy in supporting their children's education, and student–teacher relationships. See Figure 2.2 for a graph depicting change in the quality of the parent–teacher relationship during and after participation in FSS as compared to the active control group. Family–school relationships, family involvement in education, and positive student–teacher relationships can have important positive impact on student achievement and social functioning (Christenson & Sheridan, 2001; Pianta, 1999). Improvements in these areas can be important in enhancing the educational outcomes of children with ADHD. Second, the effect sizes for homework performance and parenting behavior are comparable to those achieved in the MTA study. This is very encouraging, as FSS, a relatively brief intervention that is likely feasible for implementation in clinics and schools, can have a similar impact as longer, more intensive psychosocial interventions. It should be noted that improvements in homework performance as a result of participation in FSS were identified using teacher report in addition to parent ratings. The MTA study examined intervention effects on homework performance solely according to parent report. See Figure 2.3 for a graph depicting teacher ratings of homework performance over time relative to the comparison group. Third, favorable outcomes were achieved even when FSS was compared to an active control condition, highlighting that key evidence-based components of FSS (e.g., positive reinforcement of targeted behavior, token economy, DRC, behavioral homework interventions), and not only the nonspecific elements of therapy, were critical in producing outcomes.

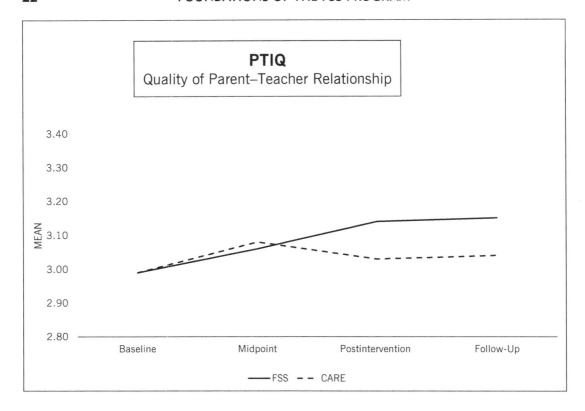

FIGURE 2.2. Between-group illustration of the change in quality of the parent–teacher relationship over the course of study participation. PTIQ; Parent–Teacher Involvement Questionnaire. The combined parent and teacher report was used in this study (Kohl et al., 2000).

What Predicts Treatment Response?

Our research has demonstrated that several factors moderate or predict response to the FSS program. Similar to other investigators (see Chronis-Tuscano et al., 2017), we have shown that the presence of elevated parental ADHD symptoms moderates the effect of FSS, although our research indicated that the effect of parental ADHD did not manifest until 3-month follow-up (Dawson et al., 2016). Families in FSS with elevated ADHD symptoms had difficulty sustaining treatment gains in the areas of child homework productivity/organization and the quality of the family–school relationship. In addition, an unexpected finding was that families in the active control condition (CARE) with elevated ADHD symptoms were able to sustain treatment gains better than those in FSS. This result suggests that elements of CARE, such as ongoing opportunities for parents to engage with each other in exploring solutions to child problems, may have been helpful in sustaining treatment gains. As such, placing greater emphasis on promoting parental self-empowerment and offering high levels of support to parents, which are key elements of motivational interviewing, may be important to promoting the sustainability of FSS outcomes.

Our research generally has shown that FSS is equally effective with families of varying demographic characteristics and children with ADHD of varying clinical presentations (Nissley-Tsiopinis et al., 2014). We did not identify any demographic or child clinical variables that moderated the effect of FSS (in comparison to CARE) on outcomes at posttreatment. However, we identified two variables that predicted treatment response for families in both FSS and CARE: presence of coexisting child anxiety and single-parent family status. Families whose child with ADHD has a coexisting anxiety disorder demonstrated more positive parenting practices after treatment than families with children who did not have this coexisting condition. The stronger response to treatment in the context of coexisting anxiety is consistent with the findings of the Multimodal Treatment of ADHD study (MTA Cooperative Group, 1999), which demonstrated that children with ADHD and a coexisting anxiety disorder generally responded better to behavioral intervention than did those without this comorbidity. In addition, our research has shown that single-parent family status was predictive of a poorer response to FSS and CARE in comparison to two-parent families. This finding supports the use of tailored BPT approaches when providing family behavioral interventions to single-parent families (Chacko et al., 2009).

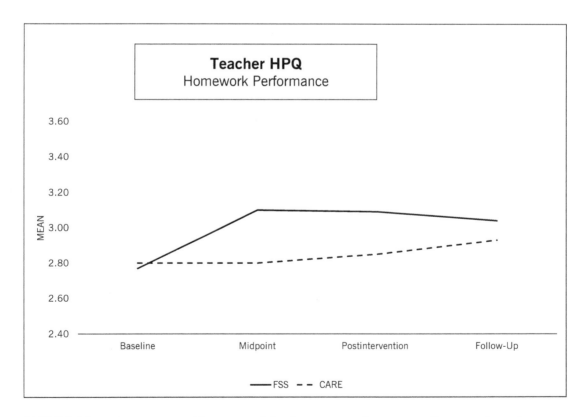

FIGURE 2.3. Between-group illustration of the change in teacher-reported homework performance over the course of study participation. HPQ; Homework Performance Questionnaire. Teacher ratings are depicted in this graph.

Does Parental Engagement in FSS Make a Difference?

In general, parental engagement in family intervention is associated with a more favorable response to treatment. Although session attendance is predictive of outcomes (Ingoldsby, 2010), quality of parental involvement in intervention has been shown to be a stronger predictor (Nix et al., 2009). A critical qualitative dimension of engagement is parental adherence to recommendations to practice strategies discussed during therapy sessions, which is typically operationalized as parental completion of between-session homework assignments. Completion of assigned homework has repeatedly been shown to be associated with a better response to treatment (Kazantzis et al., 2010; Rooney et al., 2018).

Our research with FSS confirms that parental engagement in intervention, including both attendance at sessions and adherence to assigned parental homework, is related to better outcomes (Clarke et al., 2015). In keeping with other studies, adherence is a much stronger predictor of response to treatment than attendance is. Adherence to assigned homework was associated with numerous favorable outcomes, including parental self-efficacy in fostering their children's education, quality of the parent–teacher relationship, positive parenting, attention and persistence during homework, and homework organization and productivity, with small to medium effect sizes. In contrast, parental attendance was associated with only one outcome, improved student academic productivity, with a small effect size.

These findings highlight the importance of encouraging parents to complete homework assignments designed for them to practice parenting strategies introduced during FSS sessions. In addition, the findings suggest the importance of incorporating strategies to promote family engagement and implementation of intervention strategies. These strategies might include assisting parents in coping with stress and managing their emotions, incorporating motivational interviewing strategies especially when discussing homework implementation, and helping parents identify ways to strengthen their social support network (Ingoldsby, 2010).

How Does FSS Work?

According to the theory of change, FSS has an effect on child outcomes by improving parenting practices and strengthening the parent–teacher collaboration. These hypothesized mediators are based on research demonstrating that a combined family–school intervention improves child performance by reducing negative, ineffective parenting practices (Hinshaw et al., 2000), and research indicating that a family–school problem-solving intervention (CBC) improves child performance by strengthening the family–school relationship (Sheridan et al., 2012, 2017). Our research has confirmed that FSS improves child performance by reducing negative, ineffective parenting (e.g., yelling, shaming, ordering the child around, and giving unclear instructions). Specifically, reductions in negative parenting appeared to explain at least in part the effect of FSS on parent-reported and teacher-reported homework performance (Booster et al., 2016).

Contrary to expectations, our research did not demonstrate that FSS's effect on homework performance was due to improvements in family–school collaboration (Booster et al., 2016). It should be noted that Sheridan and colleagues' research on CBC was conducted in schools, whereas our research to date has examined FSS as a clinic-based, school-linked intervention. Providing FSS in schools may afford more opportunities to strengthen family–school collaboration that might lead to improved homework performance. In addition, our research compared FSS to an active control condition that was quite effective in improving the quality of the family–school relationship and homework performance. In contrast, CBC was compared to a treatment-as-usual condition. The comparator used in studies of FSS provided a tough test of the effectiveness of this intervention, which may have produced conservative estimates of its effectiveness and reduced the likelihood of demonstrating mediation through strengthening of the family–school relationship.

CONCLUSION

This chapter provided an overview of the theoretical and empirical foundation for FSS. Behavioral, social learning, attachment, ecological systems, and self-determination theories provide the theoretical underpinnings for the program. Evidence-based strategies drawn from behavioral parent training, behavioral homework intervention, classroom behavioral intervention, and motivational interviewing, as well as strategies to support parental coping and organization, are core components of FSS. Our research has shown that FSS is:

- Acceptable to parents, teachers, and children
- Feasible for clinicians to implement
- Effective in reducing parents' use of negative parenting strategies, improving the family–school relationship, and improving child homework performance
- More effective when parents complete between-session assignments and practice skills learned in sessions

The remaining chapters provide details about how to prepare for FSS sessions, how to conduct each of the sessions, and how to evaluate family progress in the program.

CHAPTER 3

Setting Up the Family–School Success Program

Implementing FSS successfully requires a thoughtful planning process. This chapter addresses a series of practical considerations when setting up the FSS program, including:

- Which children and families are appropriate for FSS?
- Can FSS be implemented successfully in schools?
- Can FSS be implemented successfully in health and mental health settings?
- How can I recruit families for the program?
- Should I offer FSS in groups or individually?
- Should children be included in the program?
- What factors should be considered in organizing groups?
- Who can provide FSS?
- Can trainees have a role in providing FSS?

WHICH CHILDREN AND FAMILIES ARE APPROPRIATE FOR FSS?

FSS has been designed for students in grades 1–5. We have found a grade-level criterion to be more useful than an age criterion. The program can be useful for younger and older students, but adaptations are needed for these populations (see Chapter 14). The program is intended for children with a diagnosis of ADHD, but it is effective with those who have elevated symptoms of the disorder even if a formal diagnosis has not been given. FSS targets children with impairments in one or more areas, including academic and homework functioning, parent–child relationships, teacher–student relationships, and behavioral disruption at home and/or in school. This program does not explicitly focus on improving peer relationships, although children with peer problems may benefit from family participation in this program.

The program can be effective with children who have a wide range of coexisting conditions. In general, children with oppositional defiant disorder and conduct disorder can benefit from this program, but those with severe conduct problems may require more intensive, multisystemic services. In a similar vein, children with internalizing symptoms generally benefit from this program, although when concerns about anxiety and depression are more pressing than concerns about ADHD, families should be referred for cognitive behavioral therapy before receiving this service (Barbaresi et al., 2020b). Further, children with mild autism spectrum disorder (ASD) can benefit from this program, although it should be made clear to parents that FSS focuses on reducing impairments related to ADHD symptoms and not those more directly associated with ASD (e.g., social communication problems). Table 3.1 describes criteria for determining whether FSS is an appropriate program for a family. This table also suggests alternative approaches for interventions for families who may benefit from something other than FSS.

> **Learning from Our Families**
>
> For FSS to be effective, parents must be ready to engage in behavior therapy. This requires that parents realize that (1) their child has a problem that needs help, (2) they as parents can play a significant role in helping their child, and (3) they are willing to make a commitment to become involved in treatment. Barriers to care that may need to be addressed prior to participation include insurance and payment issues, scheduling concerns, child care issues, parent perceptions about the stigma of having ADHD and being involved in treatment, and lack of social support to pursue care. In addition, it is critical for parents to believe that care will be offered in a manner that is culturally humble and respectful.

TABLE 3.1. Criteria for Determining Whether FSS Is an Appropriate Intervention

FSS is well-suited for . . .	Other treatments might be better for . . .
Children in first through fifth grade (and younger children with minor adaptations)	Children in sixth grade or above (although FSS can be appropriate with adolescents with substantive adaptations; see Chapter 14)
Children with ADHD or elevated symptoms	Children without ADHD or elevated symptoms
Children with mild/moderate co-occurring conditions	Children with more severe co-occurring conditions: • Severe conduct problems (refer for multisystemic services) • Severe internalizing problems (refer for cognitive behavioral therapy) • Moderate to severe ASD (refer for intervention using applied behavior analysis)
Children with impairment in: • Academic or homework performance • Parent–child relationship • Student–teacher relationship • Behavior difficulties at home or school	Children with primary impairment in: • Peer relationships (refer for individualized family behavior therapy and school-based interventions)

CAN FSS BE IMPLEMENTED SUCCESSFULLY IN SCHOOLS?

Given the focus on family–school relationships and educational performance, FSS is well suited for delivery in schools. Delivery of FSS in schools by school-based practitioners presents several unique opportunities to address key components of the program. First, practitioners who are based in the school will have specific knowledge and understanding of available school-based resources to support youth and families coping with ADHD. This might allow for tailoring of the homework and classroom-focused intervention strategies that could increase feasibility and contextual fit. Additionally, delivery of FSS in schools might allow for enhanced consultation with teachers and support for family–school collaboration utilizing a school-based conjoint behavioral consultation model (Sheridan & Kratochwill, 2007).

Although implementation of FSS in schools comes with clear advantages related to collaboration with teachers, there are several important considerations when offering FSS in schools. First, it is important that practitioners attend to privacy issues. As discussed later in this chapter, a discussion of privacy with the group is very helpful at the outset. Given that families in groups offered in schools are much more likely to know one another than when groups are offered in clinical settings, attention to this issue is especially important.

Second, delivery of FSS in schools might present challenges related to financial sustainment. If a school-based practitioner is able to offer the program as part of typical job responsibilities (e.g., a school psychologist or school counselor), there may be fewer issues related to billing than if the program is offered by a practitioner based in a health setting or mental health agency. That said, increasingly there are mechanisms for school-based mental health clinicians to bill for services offered in school settings (Pennotti et al., 2022). We recommend that school-based practitioners interested in offering FSS familiarize themselves with billing mechanisms that might be available to support financial sustainment of the program. Additionally, offering FSS in schools may pose unique scheduling challenges. Providing services during the school day may be more convenient for school providers, and it might be feasible to include students in sessions during the school day, but these sessions may not be feasible for most caregivers to attend. Alternatively, evening sessions may be more feasible for families but more difficult for school providers to sustain.

CAN FSS BE IMPLEMENTED SUCCESSFULLY IN HEALTH AND MENTAL HEALTH SETTINGS?

FSS is highly appropriate for delivery in health and mental health organizations, and our team has had considerable experience delivering the program in these settings. In health and mental health settings, there is generally a well-established infrastructure for protecting family privacy and billing for mental health services through private and/or public payers. A potential disadvantage is that it may be challenging for practitioners to engage in consultation with school professionals; however, videoconferencing technology can be useful in mitigating this challenge. In addition, in-person services may be less convenient for families to obtain in health and mental health clinics located outside their community as opposed to in schools situated in their neighborhood. It is also feasible to offer FSS in other settings, such as primary care practices, private practices, and virtually. Chapter 14 discusses considerations for offering FSS in alternative venues.

HOW CAN I RECRUIT FAMILIES FOR FSS?

Recruitment strategies may vary depending on where the intervention will be delivered. When offered in school settings, referrals might originate from members of student support teams or multidisciplinary teams, nurses, teachers, or administrators. School mental health professionals (e.g., school psychologists, counselors, social workers) might also be aware of children and families who could benefit from participation in FSS. Additionally, parents might self-refer if they become aware of the availability of the program. Further, we recommend that pediatric primary care providers in the community be informed about the program and given specific information about how to make a referral.

Another useful way of recruiting families in schools is to provide workshops targeted for the parents of children with attention and organization difficulties. During the workshop the presenter can inform parents about the program and basic eligibility criteria for participation. In addition, it may be useful to recruit by distributing flyers in newsletters, by email, by text, or on social media platforms used by schools and/or districts. Suggestions for recruiting families when FSS is offered in primary care and private practice settings are described in Chapter 14.

If the intervention is delivered in health or mental health settings, referrals may originate from members of the clinical team (e.g., ADHD clinic, outpatient mental health service, medical practice), including professionals from multiple disciplines. In addition, giving presentations in the community to groups such as local chapters of Children and Adults with Attention-Deficit/Hyperactivity Disorder (CHADD) may be a useful recruitment strategy. Clinicians offering FSS might choose to create recruitment letters or flyers to share with colleagues and to distribute to potentially interested families. Chapter 14 describes additional strategies for recruiting families if FSS is delivered in primary care practices or private practices.

SHOULD I OFFER FSS IN GROUPS OR INDIVIDUALLY?

FSS was developed for implementation in group settings, and there are numerous advantages to providing BPT programs like FSS in a group format:

1. Parents usually benefit from the suggestions and support of other parents.
2. Group treatment is an effective method to increase the number of families served given the large volume of families who need services.
3. Group treatment may be more affordable for families in some regions.

There are challenges associated with group treatment, however, including:

1. There may be a lack of flexibility in scheduling (groups are generally scheduled on the same day and time each week).
2. If the intent is to bill third-party payers, practitioners should be aware that insurance providers may not cover multifamily group therapy without the child present, which can result in a significant financial burden for many families.
3. Some parents are not comfortable sharing with other parents in a group setting.

Assuming group care is acceptable and affordable for families, there are additional questions to consider when deciding whether a family can be treated more effectively in group or individualized care. One consideration is the complexity and severity of the child's condition(s) and level of impairment. Families of children with moderate to severe levels of oppositionality and conduct problems generally benefit from more individualized care. Children with milder variations of ASD have been treated effectively with FSS, but the focus is on treating symptoms and impairments related to the child's ADHD and not social communication difficulties associated with ASD. If two or more caregivers intend to participate in the program, a major question is whether the parents or caregivers can communicate effectively with each other to address important educational, developmental, and health issues for the child. If the parents have significant difficulty with communication, an individualized approach to therapy is strongly recommended. See Chapter 14 for suggested adaptations to FSS when delivering the program in individualized family sessions.

> **Learning from Our Families**
>
> It is important to consider parental views about receiving care in a group format. Parents may be reluctant to express their thoughts about being in a group, and some have concerns about whether they will be understood and accepted by other parents. In some cases, these concerns may be influenced by their history of marginalization and discrimination based on race/ethnicity, religion, sexual orientation, gender identity, and other factors. It is difficult to know about these factors at the time of referral and screening, but practitioners and supporting staff need to be sensitive to these issues and work actively to reduce barriers that might reduce access to and engagement in care.

SHOULD CHILDREN BE INCLUDED IN FSS?

Involving children in BPT programs like FSS is generally a good idea. Parents usually prefer that their children to be involved in therapy sessions. Although parent training not including children in sessions is effective, there is some evidence that involving children in therapy may lead to better outcomes (Webster-Stratton & Hammond, 1997). Further, involving children in group programs may reduce the cost to families for this service, given that multifamily group therapy with children present and group therapy with children are covered by insurance companies in many regions of the United States, and group intervention without children present may not be a covered service. At the end of each of the chapters describing FSS sessions (Chapters 5–13), we have included a guide for how to involve children in the session.

Despite these advantages, there are numerous challenges to involving children in FSS when offered in a group format. First, additional personnel may be needed when conducting group programs including children, because it is often advantageous for parents and children to meet separately for some components of the program. Further, it is useful to have additional staff available to provide coaching to parents and their children when practicing strategies during the session. Second, additional space may be needed for parents and children to meet separately when indicated. Third, additional time is needed to organize sessions and prepare staff when children are involved in sessions. Involving trainees can be a useful strategy to increase the number of personnel available to provide the service without significantly increasing financial costs. However, involving trainees requires substantial time and effort from practitioners to provide training and supervision, and many practitioners might not have established partnerships with training programs to identify qualified trainees.

WHAT FACTORS SHOULD I CONSIDER IN ORGANIZING GROUPS?

Planning for a cohort of families to receive FSS should be done carefully, and numerous factors need to be considered. First, practitioners need to decide whether services will be provided in person or via telehealth. There is increasing evidence that BPT can be provided feasibly and effectively using telehealth (Fogler et al., 2020), and there can be advantages to telehealth service delivery with regard to improving access to care for some families. See Chapter 14 for suggestions for delivery via telehealth. Although insurance payers increasingly are reimbursing for telehealth service delivery, reimbursement for telehealth is still evolving. Practitioners offering services via telehealth should keep this in mind. In addition, some families, especially those who are marginalized by low socioeconomic status and challenges with internet connectivity, may not have reliable access to services through telehealth. Further, in-person care may have advantages related to promoting family engagement and supporting parent implementation of assigned homework.

> **Learning from Our Families**
>
> Scheduling FSS can sometimes be a challenge. We recommend weekly meetings and have found the best time for group sessions is typically in the late afternoon or early evening. However, this can be a challenging time for families because they may be transitioning from work, preparing meals, and supporting children with homework at this time. A unique challenge in organizing groups is that parents must be available at a particular time each week and there is limited opportunity for scheduling flexibility.

Another consideration is scheduling at different times of the year. We have found the best time to initiate FSS is the end of August through the middle of April, to ensure children are in school and families will benefit from the focus on family–school collaboration and homework issues. Program modifications are needed when offering FSS at the end of the school year and during the summer when students may not be getting homework assignments or attending school. See Chapter 14 for recommended modifications when offering FSS when school is not in session.

Finally, it is important to verify the method of payment parents will use for the service and obtain informed consent from families for the service at the outset, which can be done electronically for telehealth care. The process of organizing groups can be time consuming, and it typically is not feasible for practitioners to do so on their own. For this reason, it is critical for practitioners to have sufficient administrative support to organize and prepare for FSS when it is provided in groups.

WHO CAN PROVIDE FSS?

FSS can be provided by mental health professionals from a range of disciplines. Apart from having the requisite credentials, it is important for practitioners to have training and experience in the following areas:

- Behavior therapy for children and families
- Delivery of interventions for the families of children with ADHD

- Family–school collaboration
- Teacher consultation
- Motivational interviewing
- Culturally humble and respectful care

The Preface, Chapters 1 and 2, and the references cited in these chapters may be helpful for practitioners who are interested in providing FSS but need additional training in one or more areas. In some cases, it may be appropriate for advanced trainees to provide FSS to families. Whenever possible, efforts should be made to involve practitioners and trainees of racial, ethnic, and cultural backgrounds that reflect the characteristics of participating families. Of course, it is essential for services rendered by trainees to be carefully supervised by licensed and/or certified practitioners. Billing and licensing regulations determine in part whether licensed practitioners need to provide care and need to be present when FSS sessions are offered by trainees.

CAN TRAINEES HAVE A ROLE IN PROVIDING FSS?

When providing FSS, there are several advantages to having trainees involved as cotherapists. First, this arrangement can provide a rich training experience, as students have repeated opportunities to observe experienced practitioners and practice delivering the intervention in a context where they can obtain extensive supervision. Second, trainees can assist in monitoring content and process fidelity to ensure the intervention is delivered in a high-quality manner. Finally, trainees can serve important roles in connecting with families individually to promote their engagement in intervention and support their implementation of FSS strategies. It should be acknowledged that involving trainees requires a substantial investment of time for training and supervision.

CONCLUSION

This chapter discussed key factors to consider in setting up the FSS program. For the program to be successful, it is necessary to engage in a thoughtful planning process, which will require input from many professionals, approval from administrative officials, and operational support from administrators. Our experience is that the program needs to be offered to three or four cohorts of families to resolve most of the operational challenges involved in implementing the program. That being said, challenges continually arise, and it is important to have a process in place to address these when they emerge.

At this point, you have most of the fundamentals you need to provide the FSS program. There is one more topic to address—how to conduct sessions to promote successful outcomes for each child and family. The next chapter discusses key considerations in conducting FSS sessions.

CHAPTER 4

Conducting Family–School Success Sessions

Preparation is key to having an effective FSS session. The program manual described in this guidebook (see Section II) provides a detailed set of guidelines about how to conduct each session. Practitioners need to carefully consider how they will address each session component in a way that promotes family engagement and empowerment. Each session in the manual suggests a series of open-ended questions and follow-up prompts that can be used to generate and guide discussions. In addition, the manual describes activities designed to actively engage families in sessions and promote their learning. Each session has one or more handouts and homework assignments. Practitioners need to have a plan to distribute these materials efficiently to parents. In this chapter, we address several key considerations in conducting FSS sessions, including:

- How can I manage time effectively?
- How can I protect family privacy and safety?
- What permissions do I need to communicate with teachers?
- How can I promote parent self-discovery and empowerment?
- How can I balance didactic presentation and group discussion?
- How can I implement FSS with fidelity and flexibility?
- What strategies can I use to promote family engagement?
- How can I work effectively with families from diverse backgrounds?
- How can I work effectively with parents who present challenges?
- What are useful ways to debrief after sessions?
- What is the best way to use the manual (presented in Section II)?

HOW CAN I MANAGE TIME EFFECTIVELY?

Managing time during FSS sessions, especially when delivered in groups, is an ongoing challenge. A key to time management is developing a plan for time allocation before the session begins. The program manual provides specific recommendations about how much time to allocate to sections within each session. Given the importance of supporting families in developing executive functioning skills, it is important to model for parents effective time management by clearly conveying time expectations and adhering to established limits. Practitioners need to manage time effectively, but not rigidly, as it is usually not advisable to abruptly curtail important discussions among families. In addition, it is important to emphasize the importance of being on time, reinforce families for being on time, start sessions on time, and end sessions on time. When a cotherapist is involved, a useful role for this individual is to monitor time carefully and provide prompts to promote effective time management. Additional considerations related to time management are included later in this chapter in the section on implementing the manual with flexibility.

HOW CAN I PROTECT FAMILY PRIVACY AND SAFETY?

An essential element of mental health care is protecting family privacy. Ensuring privacy is more challenging when services are offered in a group versus individually. With group care, the responsibility for protecting privacy is not only borne by the practitioner; it is shared with all families participating in the program. We inform parents at the outset that we as practitioners are mandated to respect family confidentiality (with limits to protect against harm to self or others), and we ask parents to do the same. We emphasize that parents can share with others the parenting strategies we discuss, but they cannot share personal information disclosed by participants during group meetings. In addition, we stress that participants need to exercise discretion in sharing family information during group sessions. We caution that parents should not reveal information that is personal and may reflect negatively on them or their family if inadvertently disclosed to others. During the first session we also inform parents about the limits of confidentiality. Consistent with patient care provided individually to families, the practitioner is mandated to take action and inform appropriate parties when there appears to be a safety risk, which might include child abuse, risk of self-harm, or risk of harm to others.

A limitation of providing mental health care in groups is that it can be challenging to assess child safety. This is particularly the case when children are not involved in the care. We recommend that all children receive at least a brief evaluation before commencing a parent group program. During the child evaluation, a practitioner should conduct a safety assessment and address any safety issues (e.g., violence toward others, suicidal ideation and/or behavior) that emerge. Subsequently, during each group session, it is emphasized that parents should inform the practitioner if they have any safety concerns about their child. In addition, we recommend that the practitioner or trainee contact families periodically by telephone to see how they are progressing with the program and give them an opportunity to disclose any safety concerns they have about their child.

WHAT PERMISSIONS DO I NEED TO COMMUNICATE WITH TEACHERS?

Promoting family–school collaboration is a major goal of FSS. The program focuses on facilitating this relationship by preparing parents for collaboration during FSS sessions, and it may at times involve direct communication with the child's teacher. Perhaps the most significant advantage of offering FSS in schools is that it is relatively easy for practitioners to communicate with children's teachers. If practitioners intend to communicate with teachers, they should adhere to relevant regulations protecting privacy. These regulations may differ depending on whether the FSS practitioner is an employee of the school (school district) or an external agency or clinical practice. There are two components of consent: (1) consent from the parent for the FSS practitioner to speak with the teacher and convey information about the child or family, including sharing that the family is enrolled in the FSS program; and (2) consent from the parent for educational professionals to share information with the FSS practitioner. The consent documents should specify the reason for releasing information and the scope of the information to be shared. FSS practitioners should explain to parents the requirement and purpose of consent and guide them through the consenting process. Schools and health/mental health agencies typically have forms available to ensure required information is collected at time of consent. Electronic survey tools may facilitate the process of obtaining information for these consent documents. It is critical for FSS practitioners to identify privacy and confidentiality regulations that apply for them in their setting and follow relevant policies and procedures.

HOW CAN I IMPLEMENT FSS TO PROMOTE PARENT SELF-DISCOVERY AND EMPOWERMENT?

Based on self-determination theory and principles of motivational interviewing, FSS places strong emphasis on creating a therapeutic context in which families can discover insights useful for their parenting and develop a sense of empowerment to implement evidence-based parenting strategies. The program has been designed to promote self-discovery and family empowerment by ensuring high-quality delivery of the program through the monitoring of five process fidelity dimensions. These are presented briefly in this chapter and described in more detail in Chapter 15.

The first process fidelity dimension is promoting active engagement of families by ensuring that all families are participating in group discussions, using open-ended questions to promote self-discovery, and using strategically delivered reflective statements to highlight important points raised by parents. The second process fidelity dimension is eliciting and strengthening change talk among parents by identifying and affirming indications that parents are moving or intending to move in the direction of favorable change or at least considering change. The third dimension is providing emotional validation by demonstrating empathy regarding the challenges of parenting a child with ADHD and encouraging parents to engage in strategies to promote self-care. The fourth dimension is promoting social and emotional support by fostering connections among parents and enabling them to learn from each other. The fifth dimension is maintaining parents' focus on FSS principles and empirically supported strategies.

HOW CAN I BALANCE DIDACTIC PRESENTATION AND GROUP DISCUSSION?

Because FSS places such a strong emphasis on promoting self-discovery and self-empowerment, most of the time during sessions is spent involving families in discussion. Each section of each session is organized around discussing a series of open-ended questions designed to identify key points for parents to understand. A major responsibility of the practitioner is to make comments that connect key points made by one parent with those raised by other parents, offer brief summaries of key points, and ask follow-up questions that challenge parents to explore the topic further.

Our experience has taught us that most parents already have a considerable amount of foundational knowledge. Our job is to build on the knowledge they have and facilitate a process for them to create knowledge and strengthen skills. A phrase we often use in training is to "trust the wisdom of the group." What we mean by this is to acknowledge how much parents already know and afford them the opportunity to be smart and teach others what they have learned and are discovering. Of course, parents vary in how much wisdom they bring to the program, but each parent has wisdom to share and collectively parents usually have a high level of wisdom.

Given the strong emphasis on group process, it can sometimes be challenging for practitioners to keep the discussion focused and emphasize parenting practices grounded in theory and empirical evidence. Several times during each session, it is important for practitioners to emphasize key points and offer a brief didactic presentation (i.e., typically no more than 2–3 minutes each). Practitioners need to be careful not to fall into the trap of giving longer didactic presentations, which may detract from the emphasis on promoting self-discovery and engagement. In fact, parents may often set practitioners up to be trapped in this way, placing the practitioner in an expert role by asking questions. **We encourage practitioners to keep track of the amount of time spent in group discussion versus didactic presentation; a simple rule of thumb is for at least 75% of the time to be spent in group discussion and modeling or practicing strategies.**

> **Learning from Our Families**
>
> It is very easy for practitioners to lapse into conducting sessions by giving a series of didactic presentations. Even experienced practitioners demonstrate this tendency. Monitor how much time families versus you are speaking during sessions. In addition, monitor what percentage of parental comments are being addressed to other parents versus you. It can help to involve a co-facilitator, such as a trainee, to help you keep track of the extent of family involvement. We believe that the amount of active family involvement in sessions is related to their degree of self-discovery and self-empowerment.

HOW CAN I IMPLEMENT FSS WITH FIDELITY AND FLEXIBILITY?

The manual for FSS (Section II) offers detailed guidelines for implementing each of the program sessions. It provides specific information about topics to be addressed, the sequence for discussing topics, key points to be highlighted, and strategies for involving parents actively in the therapeutic process. The manual was designed to be comprehensive and in-depth, keeping in mind that practitioners in training and those without experience in providing group BPT may benefit from having detailed information about what to do and how to do it. In general, it is recommended that practitioners provide sessions and sections within sessions in the recommended sequence, because each section builds on the previous one.

Although we suggest practitioners adhere to the basic structure and sequence of sessions, it is important for practitioners to implement the program with flexibility. The manual suggests open-ended questions to ask to elicit discussion, but practitioners are encouraged to phrase questions in a way that is comfortable for them. In addition, the manual offers recommendations for exercises to use to promote family engagement, but practitioners have latitude to adapt exercises or substitute these for alternative methods of conveying key points, teaching strategies, and offering parents opportunities for practice.

The manual also offers guidelines for how much time to spend on each section. Timelines are included as suggestions that may be useful in managing time and keeping sessions organized. Some sessions—in particular Sessions 3, 5, and 8—are relatively dense, and timelines may be useful to keep the session moving and ensuring that sections are covered. However, practitioners are encouraged to use their discretion in allocating time to sections.

> **Learning from Our Families**
>
> At times it is advisable for parents to spend more time than recommended discussing a topic, especially if parents are highly involved connecting with and supporting each other. In addition, at times it might be useful to extend the time for role play or practice during the session. Practitioners need to keep in mind that if they extend the time for one section, they will need to make up the time later in the session so that the meeting can end on time.

WHAT STRATEGIES CAN I USE TO PROMOTE FAMILY ENGAGEMENT?

The success of the program depends in part on the extent to which families attend sessions, participate actively, and complete between-session homework assignments. Our research has demonstrated that completion of homework assignments is especially related to improvements in parenting practices and child outcomes (Clarke et al., 2015; Morris et al., 2019). The main approach for promoting family engagement is attending to the process fidelity dimensions of implementation, particularly ensuring all families are actively involved in sessions, feel emotionally validated as parents and persons, and feel connected with other participating parents.

Another strategy we use is to continually emphasize the importance of completing homework assignments. When homework is given, practitioners are encouraged to explain the assignment thoroughly and acknowledge challenges that might arise with implementation. During the following session, a significant portion of time is spent discussing homework completion, identifying barriers to implementation, and discussing strategies to address barriers. In addition, practitioners are trained to identify and affirm any movement in the direction of change, including efforts to complete homework assignments.

> **Learning from Our Families**
>
> Sometimes when parents have not practiced parenting strategies at home, they might say, "I did not have time to do the homework, but I thought about it." In these cases, we recommend the practitioner focus on the parent's efforts to improve and affirm the parent by saying something like, "It is great that you took the time to think about the assignment and think about ways to implement the strategy with your child." When we provide FSS in groups, we usually contact families by phone at various points during the program (i.e., two to three times). The main purpose of these contacts is to promote family engagement and support parents with the implementation of strategies at home. Another benefit of these contacts is to give parents an opportunity to connect individually with the practitioner to share observations that may not be appropriate for group discussion. Opportunities to connect in this way may reveal concerns parents have about the program or group, giving the practitioner a chance to make accommodations to promote family engagement.

An additional strategy is to involve a professional or paraprofessional who focuses primarily on promoting family engagement and supporting families in overcoming barriers to care and implementing FSS strategies at home. These individuals have been referred to by various terms, such as *community health partner, care manager,* and *patient navigator.* It may be especially important to involve a community health partner when the practitioner(s) providing FSS do not share the cultural backgrounds of family participants. In these cases, the community health partner may help to serve as a cultural broker to ensure families view the intervention as meaningful and appropriate for addressing their concerns (Power et al., 2014).

HOW CAN I WORK EFFECTIVELY WITH FAMILIES FROM DIVERSE BACKGROUNDS?

Each family member who participates in FSS has a unique background that influences their receptivity to the program and responsiveness to the practitioner and other families in the group. For the program to be effective, practitioners need to work with each parent in a culturally humble manner, understanding how the parent is culturally unique; what aspects of their identity, family constellation, and cultural background are especially important to them; and how these factors may influence their perspective of FSS strategies.

> **Learning from Our Families**
>
> It is common for parents to question the FSS principle that parents should provide positive feedback to their children at least four times more frequently than corrective feedback (i.e., four-to-one approach). Families, especially those marginalized by race/ethnicity and low-income status, have shared they cannot take the risk of being so positive with their children. The parents may have learned it is important to use frequent, salient, corrective feedback to enforce child compliance with rules established to protect their children from harm. In these situations, it is important for the practitioner to understand the perspective of parents and work within the framework presented. An approach we have often used is to discuss the importance of balancing a positive and restrictive approach, instead of insisting the parent use a four-to-one approach.

Working with parents in groups can present unique challenges to providing services in a culturally humble way. It is important for practitioners to be aware of how each parent views the group and relates to others in the group. For example, in one group we observed that a single parent of minoritized background was quiet in a group with mostly White, two-parent families. In addition, parents who are LGBTQ+ may be uncomfortable in a group in which they perceive the other parents to be heterosexual or cisgender. When a practitioner perceives that a participant may be from a marginalized background, it is important for the practitioner to be especially conscious of facilitating connections with other parents in the group.

> **Learning from Our Families**
>
> When a parent is not actively engaged and not connecting with other parents, it is important for practitioners to question whether cultural factors or characteristics of the parent's identity may be contributing to a sense of isolation or marginalization. Arranging time to speak with this parent after a session or between sessions by phone may be helpful in identifying factors that may be contributing to isolation and potential strategies for addressing the issue.

HOW CAN I WORK EFFECTIVELY WITH PARENTS WHO EXPERIENCE CHALLENGES DURING FSS SESSIONS?

Practitioners often provide care to parents who experience challenges that interfere with their ability to fully engage in the program. These challenges may be due to a broad range of issues, including the trauma history of the parent, the attention and organization skills of the parent, and the context in which care is provided. In a group intervention, it is typical for at least one family to have such difficulties. It is important to find ways to respond to parents to increase the likelihood they will achieve favorable outcomes and minimize the possibility the challenges they experience will have a detrimental effect on others. Table 4.1 describes different types of challenges and proposed strategies for providing support.

WHAT ARE USEFUL WAYS TO DEBRIEF AFTER SESSIONS?

Taking some time for debriefing after each session is useful in evaluating progress and preparing for the next session. Completing the content and process fidelity checklists after the session is a useful strategy for guiding self-evaluation. Rating the content fidelity checklist may reveal that a component of the session was not sufficiently addressed and needs to be highlighted during the next session. Rating the process fidelity form may reveal that one or more process dimensions of intervention delivery may need to be addressed. For example, a self-evaluation may indicate that one or more parents were not actively involved in the session and additional strategies are needed to promote the engagement of these families. Alternatively, the session may have included more didactic presentation than recommended or the discussion may have veered off course at times and more redirection may be needed. In addition, the self-review could reveal that parents were spending too much time commiserating about feeling stuck, which might suggest this process could have been interrupted sooner, greater emphasis could have been placed on affirming parents for their efforts to change, and more discussion was needed to identify beginning signs of progress in positive parenting.

TABLE 4.1. Examples of Challenges That May Arise during FSS Sessions and Strategies to Provide Support

Type of challenge	Description	Strategies to support
Parent is disorganized	Struggles with organization, time management, planning; might be late to sessions, forgets between-session homework	• Affirm parent efforts to improve organization, time management, and planning • Consider having an individual discussion to support problem solving • Invite others to share effective strategies to improve organization, time management, and planning
Parent rambles during sessions	Overly talkative during sessions; comments are often disorganized and tangential	• Listen very carefully • Respectfully insert yourself in the conversation • Highlight key points made by the parent • Invite others to comment about a key point made by the parent
Parent is often skeptical	Questions the rationale for or effectiveness of recommended strategies; makes yes-but statements	• Take the questions seriously • Affirm the parent's openness to even consider a different approach • Roll with resistance • Affirm any movement toward change including efforts to try the strategy
Parent seems discouraged	Frustrated or disappointed about limited change in child outcomes; feels "stuck"	• Express empathy • Normalize the situation, indicate how common it is to feel stuck • Emphasize the importance of foundational strategies (Child's Game, Catch Child Being Good) • Point out successes (e.g., change in parenting practices even if child behavior has not yet improved)
Parent seems depressed	Displays depressed mood and pessimism; conveys little or no confidence that strategies will work	• Consider having an individual discussion about parental coping • Consider a referral to individual instead of group treatment • Explore option of adult treatment for depression, if possible • Refer to Chronis-Tuscano et al. (2020) for strategies
Parent does not follow through with recommendations	Frequently does not complete between-session homework	• Affirm movement toward change (e.g., parent intent to do homework, any efforts to perform assignments) • Explore challenges to implementation and engage in problem solving • Consider cultural issues; understand the parent's framework for parenting
Parents appears to be stressed out	Feels burdened; has difficulty being positive with children, implementing strategies	• Express empathy • Give other parents an opportunity to respond and offer support • Emphasize the importance of self-care • Encourage parent to connect with support network

(continued)

TABLE 4.1. *(continued)*

Type of challenge	Description	Strategies to support
Parent is very quiet	Talks very little during sessions; degree of engagement in sessions is not clear	• Try to understand the reasons the parent is quiet • Get to know the parent—talk after group, set up a separate time to talk • Consider cultural factors that might be contributing • Make eye contact, use body language to encourage responsiveness
Parent blames another caregiver in the family	Makes comments during group sessions that are critical of partner or other caregiver within the family	• Try to keep the focus on being accountable for one's own actions • Speak to the caregiver outside of session to understand family dynamics • Refer for individualized care, if needed

Our team often includes one or more trainees in psychology, counseling, child psychiatry, and developmental and behavioral pediatrics when offering FSS. When trainees are included in sessions, debriefing after sessions can be a highly valuable training experience. We recommend that the supervisor highlight at least one way in which each practitioner and trainee has been effective in delivering the intervention. Completing the fidelity checklists together can also be a highly effective training strategy as well as method for preparing for the next session.

WHAT IS THE BEST WAY TO USE THE FSS MANUAL?

Section II presents the manual for the FSS program. In these chapters we describe the agenda for each session, materials needed, process variables to consider in conducting the session, and goals for the session. As discussed previously, FSS places a strong emphasis on creating a context that provides opportunities for self-discovery and self-empowerment. To accomplish this purpose, practitioners are guided to address key goals of each session by engaging parents in a dialogue. Throughout the manual we suggest open-ended questions that can be used by practitioners to guide the discussion. In addition, we describe important points to highlight when addressing each goal. **The task of the practitioner is to ask good open-ended questions, listen attentively and strategically, affirm parents for participating and connecting with each other, and guide the discussion in a direction that will enable parents to come to key insights about parenting.** The application of motivational interviewing strategies is essential to promote self-discovery and self-empowerment. Careful consideration of the five process dimensions for implementing FSS will guide practitioners in using these strategies.

When conducting sessions in an inductive, conversational manner, an ongoing challenge is to manage time effectively. The manual suggests time limits to address the goals of each session. Practitioners are advised to use suggested time limits as a guide and not to apply these rigidly. It is important to balance content fidelity with process fidelity. We strongly recommend a balanced approach, as indicated by scores of 90% or higher for content fidelity and 3.5 or higher (scale of 1–4) for process fidelity (see Chapter 15 for an in-depth description of assessing fidelity).

Based on research that parental completion of between-session assignments is associated with better outcomes, FSS places strong emphasis on parental completion of assignments. The manual in Section II describes one or more assignments for parents to complete in preparation for the next session. All of these assignments are contained in Appendix A. At the end of many of these assignments, parents are asked to identify barriers to completing the assignment (i.e., implementing the parenting strategy) and potential solutions for addressing each barrier. Throughout the manual, there are prompts for practitioners to support families in the consistent implementation of program strategies.

Numerous challenges arise in providing FSS with families of varying levels of parenting skills, diverse cultural backgrounds, unique personalities, and different levels of impairment due to mental health issues (ranging from minimal to relatively severe). Throughout the manual we have inserted suggestions (i.e., Pro Tips) based on our experience for addressing challenges that commonly arise in implementing FSS with a diverse population of families.

NEXT STEPS

At this point you have the foundational knowledge needed to provide FSS. You have an understanding of the purpose and content of the program (Chapter 1); you know the goals and components of the program and you understand the theoretical and empirical foundation of the program (Chapter 2); you have considered how to set up the program (Chapter 3); and you have reflected on how to conduct sessions (Chapter 4). If you are not sure you are ready to proceed, we recommend that you reread the foundational chapters and/or consult with a colleague or supervisor. Keep in mind that no one is completely ready to provide a program like FSS before doing so. Practitioners typically need to provide the program several times to feel comfortable with intervention delivery and addressing the operational issues involved. You will become more competent and confident as you deliver the program more often. Section II (Chapters 5–13) contains the manual for the program. We strongly encourage you to review the entire manual carefully before offering the program. In addition, practitioners should study each session chapter extremely carefully before implementing the session with families.

SECTION II

THE FAMILY–SCHOOL SUCCESS MANUAL

The next nine chapters describe the FSS program manual. Each chapter includes session outlines and content for the practitioner to cover during the session, group process components and reminders, key questions to support parents on their path of self-discovery, and homework assignments. Each chapter of the program manual follows the same format:

- A brief outline of the main agenda items to cover during the session with suggestions about the amount of time to spend on each agenda item
- Materials needed for the session (including handouts and homework worksheets)
- Session process reminders
- Review of homework assigned at the end of the preceding session
- Guidance for session content organized by goals
- Homework assignments for parents to complete between sessions

To help the practitioner maintain a balance of session content and attending to group engagement and process, each section of a session is organized by providing goals and subgoals. Each subgoal includes examples of open-ended questions designed to engage parents in active discussion of specific key points. The practitioner is encouraged to use the questions provided, as well as include additional questions that support parents with understanding and integrating concepts and skills.

Each session also includes several "Pro Tips." Pro Tips represent our "lessons learned" while conducting FSS over the years. Many Pro Tips summarize guidance when working with families of diverse backgrounds, as well as addressing common challenges that may arise during sessions. We hope sharing what we have learned by working with families in the FSS program will make it easier to successfully conduct sessions.

For practitioners including children in their FSS sessions, each program manual chapter includes an outline for a child group session. The child group sessions are also organized by goals for the practitioner to accomplish with the children. Additionally, the Session 1 child group outline includes a description of group rules and a positive reinforcement point system for child group practitioners to use to support children in maintaining appropriate behavior during each session. We also include a prompt for a snack break during each session and recommend that practitioners consult with the parents of the children in the group about providing snacks (i.e., possible concerns about dietary restrictions and food allergies). Finally, each child group session concludes by engaging the children in playing a game to help make the group experience enjoyable.

CHAPTER 5

FSS Session 1
Introduction to the Family–School Success Program

Session 1 Agenda

1. Welcome families, introductions, and establish relationships among parents and program staff. (15 minutes)
2. Introduce program goals, expectations, and "Big Ideas." (20 minutes)
3. Review of ADHD and its relation to behavior and academic performance. (15 minutes)
4. Discuss the importance of family involvement in education. (15 minutes)
5. Introduce positive attending strategies. (20 minutes)
6. Assign homework and identify practice supports for consistent implementation. (5 minutes)

Materials Needed

- Handout—*Welcome to Family–School Success*
- Handout—*FSS Session Schedule*
- Handout—*FSS "Big Ideas"*
- Handout—*FSS Theory of Change*
- Handout—*Attention-Deficit/Hyperactivity Disorder—Basic Facts*
- Handout—*Attention Grid: Adult Attention as a Consequence*
- Handout—*Catch Them Being Good*
- Handout—*Homework—Noticing Positive/Desired Behavior*

- Name tags and markers
- Release of information forms for parents to provide permission to contact schools
- Dry-erase markers (to post agenda on whiteboard with time limits for each section if in-person session)

Session Process Reminders

1. Focus on using open-ended questions.
2. Practice reflective listening throughout the session to highlight and build on key points.
3. Validate emotions parents are experiencing related to their parenting.
4. Affirm parents for any effort or movement in the direction of change and implementation of recommended strategies.
5. Support all parents in participating, but avoid putting anyone on the spot.
6. Facilitate the group interacting with each other, rather than just the clinician(s).
7. Keep the group focused on session goals and refocus the discussion if it becomes tangential.

Goal 1—Welcome families, introductions, and establish relationships among parents and program staff. (15 minutes)

The goal of this section is to establish rapport and create an atmosphere in which parents feel relaxed and are willing to share their ideas and experiences. As a way to encourage parents to look for the positive in their children, we recommend that parents indicate one or more things they really appreciate about their child.

1.a. *Each member of the clinical staff introduces themselves (state name, role in the program, and experience treating children with ADHD).*

1.b. *Ask each family to introduce themselves and their children.*
- "Please tell us your name, your child's name and grade level, and something you really appreciate about your child."

Goal 2—Introduce program goals, expectations, and "Big Ideas." (20 minutes)

Helping parents understand their goals for the program is an important component of building and maintaining engagement. It is also important to describe what parents can expect by participating in the program. Additionally, many parents enter FSS after experiencing considerable challenges with their child's behavior at home and school, so it is essential that FSS is introduced in a manner that instills hope.

Session 1: Introduction to the FSS Program

2.a. *Initiate a discussion about parents' goals for participation in FSS.* This discussion should help parents identify what they hope to accomplish during the program.
- "What goals do you have for participating in this program?"
- "What do you hope to accomplish through this program?"

2.b. *Describe FSS program expectations.* Highlight the importance of active participation in group discussions and consistent completion of between-session homework assignments. If it is feasible to contact parents by phone periodically during the program, distribute a contact list and ask parents to indicate their name, phone number, and the best times to contact them during the week. Emphasize confidentiality with the parents and the expectation that parents will not discuss other families' problems and issues outside of FSS sessions. Distribute handouts *Welcome to Family–School Success* and *FSS Session Schedule.*

> **Pro Tip**
>
> Phone contact with parents between sessions may only be feasible if the clinician has trainees who can assist with this task. Secure electronic communications may be more feasible, when appropriate.

2.c. *Emphasize how important it is for parents to inform clinicians if they have concerns about the safety of their child.* Point out to parents that they can speak with you after the session if they have safety concerns. In addition, if you are able to speak with parents by phone between sessions, this provides an opportunity for them to discuss safety issues.

2.d. *Introduce and initiate a discussion about the FSS "Big Ideas."* This discussion focuses on the three foundational principles of FSS: (1) cultivating a strong parent–child relationship, (2) developing a home environment that supports learning and promotes educational success, and (3) building a collaborative parent–teacher relationship that supports the child's educational growth. Distribute the handout *FSS "Big Ideas"* and engage parents in discussion about how the "Big Ideas" connect with program goals.
- "Big Idea #1 is the importance of strengthening the parent–child relationship. How can a strong parent–child relationship be helpful to your child?"
- "Big Idea #2 is establishing a home environment that supports learning and promotes educational success. What are some ways that parents can create a home that leads to success at school?"
- "Big Idea #3 is developing a collaborative parent–teacher relationship to support a child's educational growth. How is the parent–teacher relationship important for the child's success at school?"

2.e. *Orient parents to the FSS theory of change.* Emphasize that FSS includes strategies to improve children's functioning at home and school. In addition, FSS addresses the need for parents to improve their organizational and emotional self-regulation skills.

2.f. *If it is feasible for a clinician to reach out to the school, obtain a release of information from parents to communicate with child's teacher/school.* The purpose of the release of information is to permit FSS clinicians to communi-

> **Pro Tip**
>
> The purpose of having a clinician connect with the school is to prepare educators for family–school collaboration. This connection may also be helpful to clinicians in coaching parents to communicate with educators.

cate with the child's teacher and inform the teacher about the family's participation in FSS. It is recommended that clinicians use HIPAA-compliant release of information forms.

Goal 3—Review of ADHD and its relation to behavior and academic performance. (15 minutes)

Parents likely will benefit from a quick review about ADHD, its causes and neurodevelopmental mechanisms, and its treatments. It is assumed that families participating in this program already have basic knowledge about ADHD, but a brief review is often helpful.

3.a. *Engage parents in a discussion of how ADHD is affecting their child's behavior and performance.* After brainstorming with parents, it is helpful to distinguish the problems into symptoms (inattention vs. hyperactivity-impulsivity); impairments in academic, social, and behavioral functioning; and coexisting conditions (e.g., oppositional defiant disorder, anxiety disorder, learning disability, autism spectrum disorder).

- "What are the challenges your child is experiencing at home and school?"
- "What impact are these problems having on your child?"

3.b. *Provide brief education about the genetics and neurobiology of ADHD as well as evidence-based treatments for this condition.* Encourage parents to read the handout *Attention-Deficit/Hyperactivity Disorder: Basic Facts* to learn more about ADHD.

- "What approaches to the treatment of ADHD are you currently using or have you tried in the past?"
- "What are the most important things you as parents can do to help your children develop into healthy, successful, and caring individuals?"

Goal 4—Discuss the importance of family involvement in education. (15 minutes)

Families may be involved in their children's education in a variety of ways (e.g., volunteering at school, communicating with the teacher about the child's educational progress, engaging in educational activities at home). It is helpful for parents to appreciate that although children learn much at school, they also learn a great deal from their parents and other family members. In addition, it is important to remember that children's educational performance and view of school is affected by the relationship between parents and teachers/school staff.

4.a. *Engage parents in a discussion about what they can do to help their children succeed in school.* Parents can promote school success by working on strengthening the relationship they have with their child, engaging in rewarding educational activities with their child in the home, and developing strong relationships with their child's teachers.

- "What do you do at home that helps your child do well in school?"
- "How does a strong family–school relationship have an impact on your child?"
- "What strategies do you use to build and maintain a strong relationship with your child's teachers?"

4.b. *Emphasize the importance of developing and maintaining a collaborative relationship between family and school.* Effective collaboration entails ongoing communication, empathy for the other, and a deep respect for the authority of each party in their respective domains (teacher at school and parent at home).

Goal 5—Introduce positive attending strategies. (20 minutes)

It is essential for parents to understand that positive attending is a foundational strategy to change their child's behavior. Parents may enter FSS expecting to learn about methods of punishment, so it is important to explain why focusing on positive attending at the outset is important before addressing punitive strategies. Distribute the handouts *Attention Grid: Adult Attention as a Consequence* and *Catch Them Being Good*. We recommend using the Attention Grid graphic as a way of stimulating discussion about positive, strategic attending and its counterpart, strategic ignoring.

5.a. *Initiate a discussion about how parents deploy their attention when parenting their child.* Refer to the *Attention Grid* during this discussion. Clinicians should make the point that parents typically pay attention to their children when they are misbehaving and not when they are behaving appropriately. By so doing, parents unwittingly reinforce behavior they want to reduce or eliminate. It may be useful for the clinician to draw the attention grid on a whiteboard to help parents understand these points.

- "How do you typically respond when your child is not following rules or not behaving appropriately?"
- "How do you typically respond when your child is following rules, playing cooperatively, and paying attention during homework?"
- "What is the impact of paying attention to your child's misbehavior?"
- "What is the impact of not paying attention to your child's appropriate behavior?"

5.b. *Continue the discussion by asking parents about the impact of ignoring children when they are engaged in inappropriate behavior.* Ignoring or strategically deciding not to pay attention to unwanted behavior will have the effect of reducing the targeted behavior. Implementing this strategy can be challenging for parents because children's behavior will often get worse before it improves. Most children have learned that escalating their misbehavior in response to ignoring is effective in getting their parents to stop ignoring and pay attention to them. It is important for parents to be persistent when using ignoring to reduce unwanted behaviors.

> **Pro Tip**
>
> Most parents need support to work through their impatience when children's misbehavior escalates in response to ignoring. It is helpful to engage parents in a discussion about what they can do to manage their frustration so they do not back down and stop ignoring.

- "What happens when you ignore your child for behaving inappropriately?"
- "Why does your child's behavior often get worse when you first use ignoring?"
- "How can you remain persistent and consistent when ignoring your child?"

Goal 6—Assign homework and identify practice supports for consistent implementation. (5 minutes)

- *Ask parents to record at least three instances when they noticed their child's desired behavior, what they did to show the child that they noticed the behavior, and their child's reaction to their positive attending.* This should be recorded on the *Noticing Positive/Desired Behavior* homework sheet.
- *Encourage parents to identify barriers to using positive attending as a response to their child's desired behavior and strategies to address each barrier.* Request that parents record this information at the bottom of the homework sheet.
- *Encourage parents to call you if any questions or concerns arise in the coming week.* Emphasize the importance of implementing the homework assignment.

Session 1 Child Group Agenda

1. Orient children to the components of FSS.
2. Define rules and expectations for the group and introduce the token reinforcement system.
3. Build group cohesion and relationships.
4. Introduce positive reinforcement.
5. Conclude session.

Materials Needed

- For token reinforcement system—stopwatch/timer (for keeping track of 15-minute intervals) and flip chart
- For Dog, Cat, Pig Game—animal picture cards, bag, blindfold (or materials for other group cohesion games)
- Name tags
- Deck of playing cards
- Crayons/markers
- Reinforcers that can be used as part of a token reinforcement system
- Snacks for snack break during session

Goal 1—Orient children to the components of FSS.

Escort children into the child therapy room after a brief, joint orientation with their parents and provide orientation to the child group sessions.

- Provide children with a rationale for the group (e.g., you and your parents are here to help make homework easier and help you do well in school).
- Review the agenda for the current session and activities, as well as a preview of future sessions' activities.
- Develop a group name with the children and write colorfully on the flip chart.

Goal 2—Define rules and expectations for the group, and introduce the token reinforcement system.

Facilitate a discussion of group rules and the purpose of having rules, and have children agree on three or four rules. Group rules should be posted so that children can see them throughout each session. After establishing the group rules, group leaders should explain the token reinforcement system ("reward system") that will be used during each session.

- Every 15 minutes, the group leaders will rate each child on how well they followed the group rules.
- The children earn 0 points if they had difficulty following all or most rules, 1 point if they followed most rules, and 2 points if they followed all group rules well.
- Children are not allowed to contest the number of points they receive. If children protest, they should be reminded that the points are not negotiable and that they can try harder to get 2 points at the next checkpoint.
- At the end of the session, the children will be allowed to choose a small (e.g., sticker), medium (e.g., fancy pencils), and a large (e.g., small toys) reward based on total number of points.
- Start timing the first 15-minute interval.

Goal 3—Build group cohesion and relationships.

After establishing group program rules and helping children understand the token reinforcement system, group leaders should facilitate the forming of relationships among children.

- Ask children to make and decorate name tags.
- Play Get to Know You Game.
  - Have everyone sit in a circle. Pass around a small bag of token reinforcement tokens/tickets and ask each child to take up to five tokens/tickets. Next, ask each child to say one thing about themselves for each token/ticket that they are holding. Each time they say something about themselves, they give one of the token/tickets to the group leader to add to their session total.
- Prepare children for the upcoming break, by explaining that all rules still apply, and describing how children will take turns going to the bathroom.

Snack Break

Continue building group cohesion by playing a game with the group. An example is the Dog, Cat, Pig Game.

- For six players (for more than six children, additional cards with other animals can be included): Create cards with an image of a dog, cat, or pig on each. Put two cards of each type of animal (dog, cat, pig) into a bag. Children draw cards out of bag, and then have to find their partner by making noises crawling on floor (while blindfolded).

Goal 4—Introduce positive reinforcement.

This goal focuses on helping children understand the concept of positive reinforcement and provides them with a foundation for their parents' increased attention to desired behavior.

- Have children take turns saying at least one positive thing about themselves. Engage children in trying to remember the positive thing children seated next to them stated.
- Ask children what things their parents think they do well and ask them how their parents should react when they do a good job.
- Ask children what things their parents think they do not do well and ask them how their parents should react when they do not do a good job.
- Ask children how they feel when their parents ignore them when they do not do a good job.

Goal 5—Conclude session.

- Engage children in a card game or art activity, according to their choice, if there is time remaining.
- Announce point totals and allow children to choose prizes. Emphasize positive behaviors displayed by each child. Do not focus on disruptive behaviors. Rather, encourage children to keep up the effort to follow rules throughout the week and at the next session.

CHAPTER 6

FSS Session 2
Strengthening Family Relationships

Session 2 Agenda

1. Review homework on positive attending and identify strategies for overcoming barriers to implementation. (25 minutes)
2. Discuss parent coping strategies to promote implementation of effective parenting strategies. (20 minutes)
3. Model Child's Game. (15 minutes)
4. Discuss the key components of Child's Game and provide opportunity for practice with clinician coaching. (25 minutes)
5. Assign homework and identify practice supports for consistent implementation. (5 minutes)

Materials Needed

- Handout—*Child's Game*
- Handout—*Child's Game Homework Sheet*
- Handouts—*FSS Theory of Change* and *Attention Grid* (both distributed in Session 1)
- Toys for modeling Child's Game (e.g., Legos, crayons/markers, paper, cars/trucks, dolls, and toy furniture)
- Timer to manage time during modeling and practicing of Child's Game
- Dry-erase markers (to post agenda on whiteboard with time limits for each section)

Session Process Reminders

1. Focus on using open-ended questions.
2. Practice reflective listening throughout the session to highlight and build on key points.
3. Validate emotions parents are experiencing related to their parenting.
4. Affirm parents for any effort or movement in the direction of change and implementation of recommended strategies.
5. Support all parents in participating and avoid putting anyone on the spot.
6. Facilitate the group interacting with each other, rather than just the clinician(s).
7. Keep the group focused on key points and refocus the discussion if it becomes tangential.

Goal 1—Review homework on positive attending and identify strategies for overcoming barriers to implementation. (25 minutes)

Facilitate families reintroducing themselves to each other. This helps group members become more comfortable with each other and is helpful if a new family joins the program after Session 1.

Collect completed homework assignments and make copies. The purpose of collecting assignments is to increase accountability and encourage consistent implementation.

Request that a parent review the discussion held in the first session on positive attending. Doing so will be helpful for any parent who did not attend that session and will serve as a useful reminder for others.

1.a. *Discuss parents' experiences with the homework assignment on positive attending.* Focus on and affirm any efforts parents have made to implement the homework assignment on positive attending.
- "How did the homework assignment go?"
- "What did you learn?"
- "What positive behaviors did you notice?"
- "What behaviors did you notice that you previously took for granted?"
- "How did you reinforce your child for performing these behaviors?"
- "What made it difficult for you to practice positive attending?"
- "What challenges did you experience?"
- "What strategies did you use to overcome any barriers?"

1.b. *Review the handout—FSS Theory of Change.* It is important to put strategies in context for the families to encourage learning. Relate the strategies back to the "Big Ideas" of the program and the theory of change.
- "What are the 'Big Ideas' of the Family–School Success program?"
- "How is the Family–School Success program designed to help your child at home and school?"

Goal 2—Discuss parent coping strategies to promote implementation of effective parenting strategies. (20 minutes)

This section focuses on how parents are coping as individuals. To be effective in implementing positive parenting strategies, it is critical for parents to have strong coping skills, including organizational strategies, self-regulation skills, and supportive relationships with other caregivers. This section provides an opportunity for parents to share what it is like for them to be parents. Encourage parents to discuss the stress they experience, the exhaustion they often feel in parenting a child with ADHD, and the guilt they may feel when they say or do something that is not helpful for their child. It is important for clinicians to listen for and reflect feelings and facilitate sharing of feelings among family members.

> **Pro Tip**
>
> It is common for parents to avoid discussing their own emotional experiences related to parenting their child with ADHD. This may be due to several factors, including the parents' desire to focus on improving their child's behavior and/or their discomfort talking about themselves. If needed, it is important to respectfully and tactfully redirect the conversation to support parents in focusing on themselves and identifying ways to improve their coping strategies.

2.a. *Acknowledge that parenting children with ADHD takes superhuman effort and organizational skills.* Engage parents in sharing strategies they use each day to keep themselves organized. Ask them to discuss how they are balancing work/school/home life, and their child's activities outside of school.

- "What organization and time management strategies do you already use in your daily lives (for work, organizing dinners, after school activities, etc.)?"
- "What other strategies might help you to parent more effectively?"

2.b. *Acknowledge that parenting can be stressful, especially when you have a child with ADHD.* Engage parents in a discussion about what it is like for them to parent a child with ADHD and maintain a positive attitude.

- "Do you ever feel misunderstood as a parent of a child with ADHD?"
- "What emotions do you experience in coping with the challenges of being the parent of a child with ADHD?"
- "What strategies do you use to control the anger, guilt, and stress you experience as a parent?"
- "How do you deal with the stress of parenting?"
- "What strategies do you use to maintain emotional balance and control?"

2.c. *Point out that being effective in parenting a child with ADHD requires that you have the support of other caregivers.* Engage parents in a discussion about how they get support from other caregivers. It is also important to recognize that there may be a range of family constellations represented in the group (e.g., single-parent households, multigenerational households, and extended family households). Emphasize to parents that positive reinforcement strategies work well with adults as well as children. Discuss with parents methods to further develop the roles of these other adults as partners in caregiving. Keep in mind that there are many ways parents can obtain support from other caregivers/household members/extended family.

- "How do you get the support you need as a parent?"
- "Whom do you contact when you need support from others?"
- "How did you work with another caregiver/family member to complete last week's homework assignment?"
- "How can you acknowledge each other's efforts?"
- "What can you do to strengthen the relationships you have with key caregivers in your child's life?"

> **Pro Tip**
>
> If a group member speaks negatively about another caregiver in their family during the session, provide an empathic statement (such as "I understand that it is often challenging to get the support of others in your family and parents often feel isolated"). Reframe the discussion to focus on what is under the parent's control and what the parent can do to improve the situation. It may also be helpful to provide this group member an opportunity to talk with the group leader after the session to further support effective collaborative parenting.

Goal 3—Model Child's Game. (15 minutes)

This section focuses on helping parents understand the rationale for Child's Game (or Special Time) and teaching the components of this strategy. The main goal of Child's Game is to strengthen the parent–child relationship. Parents can build the relationship with their child through frequent and ongoing opportunities to engage in child-directed play. Stronger parent–child relationships will help the child to control behavior and emotions better, and relate to teachers and peers more effectively.

3.a. *Discuss with parents why it is important to spend time playing with their children.*
- "What are some positive effects of spending time playing with your child?"
- "How can parent–child play support improvements in behavior?"

3.b. *Engage parents in talking about how they play with their child.*
- "What are some ways that you play with your children?"
- "How do you play with your child(ren) in a manner that shows how much you appreciate them?"
- "What are some strategies you want to be conscious of when you play with your child?"

3.c. *Model parent behavior when engaged in parent–child play.* Explain to parents that you are initially going to demonstrate ways to play with their child that are NOT RECOMMENDED. The initial model, which lasts about 2 minutes, should include examples of Child's Game being conducted incorrectly, which will illustrate the "Do not Use or DON'Ts" of Child's Game (see Goal 4 for examples). The lead clinician (acting in the role of parent) and clinical assistant or trainee (acting in the role of child) will engage in a Child's Game activity while the parents have an opportunity to observe. If a clinical assistant or trainee is not available to assist the clinician, a parent can be recruited to serve in the role of child.
- "What did you observe the parent doing in this role play that was not helpful?"
- "What effect did these play strategies have on the child?"

Following this, explain to parents that you are going to demonstrate play strategies that are RECOMMENDED, that is, the "DO" skills of Child's Game. Model Child's Game using the PRIDE skills described in Goal 4.

- "What did you observe the parent doing in this role play that was helpful?"
- "What effect did these play strategies have on the child?"

Goal 4—Discuss the key components of Child's Game and provide opportunity for practice with clinician coaching. (25 minutes)

Following the modeling of Child's Game, point out to parents the rules to follow (DOs and DON'Ts) of Child's Game. After that, give parents an opportunity to practice this set of skills. Distribute the handout *Child's Game*.

4.a. *Point out to the parents that Child's Game is an opportunity for parents and children to spend time together for approximately 10–15 minutes per day.* Child activities during play will vary substantially depending on the age of the child. Indicate that almost any child activity can be turned into Child's Game if parents are attentive to their child, follow their child's lead, and continually show appreciation for their child. The child should: (1) lead the interaction, (2) select the activity, and (3) determine the course of the activity/play.

4.b. *Review the rules of Child's Game.* Highlight the importance of following the child's lead and making sure the child is the center of attention.

- Inform parents of the "DO" Skills of Child's Game by referring to PRIDE skills.
  - **Praise** the child for "OK behaviors."
  - **Reflect** what the child says.
  - **Imitate** the child's play.
  - **Describe** what the child is doing (The parent should act as a "commentator" or "sportscaster" during the game. This is an opportunity to provide frequent positive reinforcement that is not contingent on meeting expectations or following adult rules/demands).
  - Communicate genuine **Enthusiasm**.
- Highlight for parents the "DON'T DO" strategies during Child's Game. Encourage parents to:
  - Refrain from giving commands or directions (remind parents that this is one of the very few times during the day when children can direct the activity and receive parental attention without adults making the rules or placing demands on the child).
  - Refrain from asking questions (explain to parents that by asking a question, we expect a response from the child, which places a demand on the child).
  - Refrain from directing the child's play.

4.c. If children do not attend the session, organize parents into pairs for role playing of Child's Game. Two caregivers from the same family can be placed in the same pair. Each parent should have an opportunity to practice being the parent and child during the role-play session. If children attend the session, give each parent an opportunity to engage in Child's Game with their child. If more than one parent in a family is present, parents can take turns playing with their child and observing. Clinicians should move about the room, observing each pair to provide feedback, with an emphasis on catching each parent using the strategy effectively.

4.d. *Engage parents in a discussion about how to implement Child's Game with their child.* Ask parents to identify potential barriers and solutions for these. If the child misbehaves during Child's Game, ignore the behavior at first. If the misbehavior continues, give a warning that the game will end if the misbehavior continues. If misbehavior persists, end the game and inform the child you will return to the game later. Establish time limits for Child's Game, so it only lasts for a reasonable period.

- "How can you implement this strategy with your child?"
- "How challenging will it be to find the time to do Child's Game?"
- "How can you adjust your schedule to find time for Child's Game?"
- "How can you use Child's Game if you only have a couple minutes to spend with your child?"
- "What should you do if your child misbehaves during Child's Game?"
- "What should you do if your child demands to extend Child's Game beyond the established time limit?"
- "Who can help you with siblings during Child's Game?"
- "How could you involve siblings in Child's Game if it is not possible to engage in this activity individually with your child?"

> **Pro Tip**
> Parents often indicate they have trouble finding time for Child's Game. Point out that a parent and child can play Child's Game at any time. The only requirement for Child's Game is for parents to have the right frame of mind, which includes emptying their thoughts, listening to their child, and affirming their child. Parents can do this when they have very little time, including driving their child around in the car and watching their child play video games.

Goal 5—Assign homework and identify practice supports for consistent implementation. (5 minutes)

- *Parent(s) (both parents, whenever relevant) and child should engage in Child's Game on at least three occasions between now and the next session.* Distribute the handout *Child's Game Homework Sheet.* Ask parents to complete the homework worksheet and consider barriers to implementation, as well as strategies to overcome the barriers.
- *Discuss the importance of consistent implementation.* Remind parents that all parents face challenges in using recommended strategies on a frequent and consistent basis.
  - Ask parents to think about their implementation of Child's Game throughout the week and consider any barriers they face with implementation (provide an example).
  - Ask parents: How could they overcome the barrier(s)?
- *Encourage parents to contact you if any questions or concerns arise in the coming week.*

Session 2: Strengthening Family Relationships

Session 2 Child Group Agenda

1. Review the group rules and token reinforcement system.
2. Continue to build group cohesion.
3. Prepare children for Child's Game.
4. Return to parent group to practice Child's Game.

Materials Needed

- For token reinforcement system—stopwatch/timer (for keeping track of 15-minute intervals) and flip chart
- Name tags
- Deck of playing cards
- Crayons/markers
- Reinforcers that can be used as part of a token reinforcement system
- Snacks for snack break during session

Goal 1—Review the group rules and token reinforcement system.

Escort children into the child therapy room after a brief, joint orientation with their parents. The first goal is to make sure the children are oriented to the group rules that were developed during the initial session and the token reinforcement system.

- Remind children of the group name they agreed on during the initial session.
- Ask children to identify rules that were identified during the initial session.
- Review how the token economy operates and ask children if they have any questions.
- Review the agenda for the current session and activities.
- Start the first 15-minute interval for the token reinforcement system.

Goal 2—Continue to build group cohesion.

Building group cohesion was an important part of Session 1. During this second group session, group leaders should continue to establish group relationships.

- Ask each child what they liked best about the first group session. Each child should be encouraged to talk about at least one thing they enjoyed.
- Ask children to share at least one thing they really like about their family. Praise children for participating. Encourage them to think of other nice things to say.

Goal 3—Prepare children for Child's Game.

The goal of this portion of the child group session is to prepare the children for the Child's Game activity that their parents will start implementing. This should include helping the children identify what they enjoy about playing with their parents and providing the children with an overview of Child's Game.

- Ask children to share some ways they enjoy playing with their parents.
- Engage children in discussion of how playing with their parents makes them feel.
- Provide children an overview of Child's Game (parents will spend 10–15 min per day engaging them in play; children get to select the activity).
- Guide children in identifying activities they can play during Child's Game.
- Prepare children for the upcoming break, by explaining that all rules still apply, and describing how children will take turns going to the bathroom.

Snack Break

Goal 4—Return to parent group to practice Child's Game.

The children will return to the parent group session to engage in practice of Child's Game with their parents.

- Prior to returning to the parent group, announce point totals and allow children to select prizes. Emphasize positive behaviors displayed by each child. Do not focus on disruptive behaviors. Rather, encourage children to keep up the effort to follow rules throughout the week and at the next session.
- After prize selection, escort children to the parent group room for practice of Child's Game with their parents.

CHAPTER 7

FSS Session 3
Understanding the Basics of Behavior Management

Session 3 Agenda

1. Review homework on practice of Child's Game with a focus on consistent implementation. (20 minutes)
2. Help parents understand and analyze antecedents and consequences of behavior. (15 minutes)
3. Educate parents about using effective ways of giving instructions to their child (antecedent strategy). (10 minutes)
4. Introduce basic consequence strategies for behavior management. (30 minutes)
5. Discuss types of reinforcers. (10 minutes)
6. Assign homework and identify practice supports for consistent implementation. (5 minutes)

Materials Needed

- Handout—*The A-B-C Model of Behavior*
- Handout—*Effective Instructions*
- Handout—*Understanding and Changing the Consequences of Behavior*
- Handout—*Using Positive Reinforcement*
- Handout—*Homework—A-B-C Worksheet*
- Handout—*Homework—Reward Menu*

- Handouts (or posters)—*FSS Theory of Change* and *Attention Grid* (both distributed in Session 1)
- Dry-erase markers (to post agenda on whiteboard with time limits for each section if in-person session)

Session Process Reminders

1. Focus on using open-ended questions.
2. Practice reflective listening throughout the session to highlight and build on key points.
3. Validate emotions parents are experiencing related to their parenting.
4. Affirm parents for any effort or movement in the direction of change and implementation of recommended strategies.
5. Support all parents in participating, and avoid putting anyone on the spot.
6. Facilitate the group interacting with each other, rather than just the clinician(s).
7. Keep the group focused on key points and refocus the discussion if it becomes tangential.

Goal 1—Review homework on practice of Child's Game with a focus on consistent implementation. (20 minutes)

Child's Game can be challenging for parents to implement for a variety of reasons. It is important to support families in sharing their experiences, as this will enable group members to learn from each other.

Collect completed homework, review, and return homework to parents. The purpose of collecting homework is to increase accountability and encourage consistent implementation. Making copies of the homework will enable the group leader to score homework completed after the session. Continue to emphasize the importance of completing homework assignments. Encourage parents to share how they receive support from other caregivers in implementing homework assignments.

1.a. *Ask families to share their experiences with Child's Game.* Ask them to describe the activity, how they participated, how they acknowledged their child's behavior during Child's Game, and how the child responded. Praise the parents for their effort in practicing Child's Game. Affirm parents for any movement in the direction of change, even if they only had time for a brief Child's Game or the activity was not as successful as they had hoped.

- "How did the homework go? What was the experience like for you?"
- "What kinds of games did you play with your child?"
- "How did your child respond?"
- "How did you modify Child's Game to work for your child?"
- "What did you find challenging?"

Session 3: Understanding the Basics of Behavior Management 63

- "What barriers to implementation did you identify?"
- "What strategies did you use to overcome the barriers?"
- "How did you manage the urge to take control of the play? What about the urge to ask questions?"
- "How did it feel for you to implement this strategy?"
- "How can you incorporate Child's Game into your daily routine?"

1.b. *Prompt parents to share ways they receive support from their partners (or other family members) in completing the homework.* Discuss how caregivers can support each other and highlight the importance of having a support system to manage ADHD.

- "How did you coordinate Child's Game practice with your partner or other family members who help with your child?"
- "What challenges did you find having more than one parent involved in practicing? What did you do to manage the challenges?"

Goal 2—Help parents understand and analyze the antecedents and consequences of behavior. (15 minutes)

This section focuses on helping parents better understand factors that contribute to a child behaving in a desirable or undesirable way. It is important for parents to differentiate between antecedents that elicit target behaviors and consequences that maintain the behaviors. Distribute the handouts *The A-B-C Model of Behavior* and *Homework—A-B-C Worksheet*.

2.a. *Discuss the A-B-Cs of child behavior.* A refers to antecedents; B refers to behaviors; C refers to consequences. Draw three columns on the whiteboard and label the columns "A," "B," and "C." Ask parents to define antecedents (A), which are events or circumstances that precede the occurrence of a behavior that increase or decrease the likelihood the behavior will occur. Antecedents are useful in behavioral change to "stack the deck" to make it more likely children will perform desired behaviors; antecedents set children up for success and make it more likely children's behavior will warrant positive reinforcement. It is also important for parents to recognize that antecedents can also make it more likely that undesired behavior will occur.

- "What circumstances or antecedents make it more likely for your child to perform undesired behaviors?"
- "What antecedents stack the deck to help your child behave in a desired way?"

2.b. *Ask parents to give examples of target behaviors (B), that is, behaviors they would like to target for change.* Parents will typically indicate behaviors for the child to perform less. Ask parents to reframe stated behaviors into actions they would like to see more often. For example, if the parent initially indicates the target behavior is not following directions, parents could reframe this behavior as "first time listening" or following directions the first time they are given. Additionally, target behaviors should require an active response from the child and pass the "dead person's test" (i.e., if a dead person can perform the behavior [stay still], then it is not an appropriate target behavior). Reframing target behaviors in this way is important because it prompts parents to look for desirable behaviors and catch their child being good.

- "What are some behaviors you would like to see increase?"
- "How can you reframe your child's problematic behaviors as behaviors you would like to see more of?"

2.c. *Ask parents to define consequences (C), that is, events that occur after target behaviors that increase or decrease the likelihood that the behavior will occur.* Help parents give examples of different types of consequences, such as positive reinforcement, ignoring, and punishment.

- "What are examples of positive reinforcement and punishment that influence your child's behavior?"
- "Can you think of alternative consequences that might also be useful? What about ignoring?"

2.d. *Engage parents in an exercise to practice applying the A-B-C model to analyze behavior.* Ask parents to think about a child behavior they would like to change. Ask one parent to indicate the behavior selected. Parents will typically identify an undesirable behavior they would like to see less of. Lead the parents through an A-B-C analysis of this behavior. Subsequently, ask the parents to reframe the target behavior into what they would like to see the child do more of. Conduct another A-B-C analysis for the target behavior they would like the child to perform more often.

Goal 3—Educate parents about effective ways of giving instructions to their child (antecedent strategy). (10 minutes)

The way that parents provide instructions or directions to their child is an important environmental event (antecedent) that can elicit behavior from their children (either desired or undesired). Properly communicated instructions have a greater chance of resulting in compliant child behavior than ineffectively issued instructions. In this section, parents will learn specific guidelines about how to communicate instructions as a key antecedent behavior management strategy.

> **Pro Tip**
>
> Parents usually have good ideas about giving instructions to their children in an effective way, even if they do not implement these strategies consistently. Try to get parents to elicit these strategies on their own.

3.a. *Help parents identify effective strategies to communicate instructions.* We recommend identifying ways NOT to give instructions before identifying effective approaches.

- "If you need your child to listen to you, what are approaches to giving instructions that would likely NOT be effective?"
- "If you need your child to listen, what are approaches to giving instructions that would be effective?"

Session 3: Understanding the Basics of Behavior Management 65

3.b. *Engage parents in an exercise of generating ways to give effective instructions.* Encourage parents to develop a list of techniques for communicating instructions clearly.

- "What are ways to give instructions that make it likely your child will listen and follow through?"

3.c. *Distribute and review the handout—Effective Instructions.* Parents are likely to generate most of the techniques on their own. Highlight for parents additional techniques they can use.

Goal 4—Introduce parents to basic consequence strategies for behavior management. (30 minutes)

This section is designed to help parents build a foundational understanding of how to apply consequences in a strategic manner to promote changes in child behavior. The discussion of consequences should be nested in the context of the A-B-C model. By so doing, parents will develop a deeper understanding of these strategies and be better able to generalize their use across situations. Distribute the handout *Understanding and Changing the Consequences of Behavior.*

4.a. *Initiate the discussion by asking parents for their ideas about positive reinforcement.* Make sure parents understand that positive reinforcement is a consequence (a *C* in the A-B-C model) and functions by increasing the likelihood that a behavior will occur again in the future.

> **Pro Tip**
>
> Parents often confuse negative reinforcement and punishment. It is often helpful for parents to understand that negative reinforcement is reinforcement, in particular it is the satisfaction you get when you are able to avoid doing something you don't want to do (e.g., avoid homework, get your parents not to follow through with a demand).

- "What is positive reinforcement?"
- "Is positive reinforcement an antecedent or consequence strategy?"
- "What is the goal of using positive reinforcement?"

4.b. *Help parents understand the difference between positive and negative reinforcement.* It is important for parents to understand that the *negative* in negative reinforcement refers to the removal of an undesirable stimulus as the result of performance of a behavior, which has the effect of increasing the probability of the behavior occurring in the future. Some examples include (1) putting on your car seatbelt (target behavior) is negatively reinforced when the reminder signal (undesired stimulus) terminates, and (2) parents buying candy at the supermarket checkout line for their whining child (target behavior) is negatively reinforced when the child stops whining (undesired stimulus). However, it should be noted that in this example the child's whining is positively reinforced. In other words, the parent is more likely to give in to the child whining in the future (due to negative reinforcement) and the child is more likely to whine in these situations (due to positive reinforcement).

- "Now that you understand positive and negative reinforcement, how are they different?"
- "Can you think of other examples of negative reinforcement?"

4.c. *Work with parents to apply the principle of negative reinforcement to better understand their child's behavior.* The goal of this portion is to help parents gain experience using the concept of negative reinforcement to understand some of the factors that maintain undesired behavior. Specifically, parents will be guided to think about how negative reinforcement is a factor in homework completion. Delaying/putting off homework (target behavior) may be negatively reinforcing to the child because it temporarily enables the child to avoid an unpleasant task. Nonadaptive behaviors may take the form of making noises, disturbing others, or playing with a pet, which serve as ways to get out of doing work.

- "How does negative reinforcement account for a child's tendency to procrastinate at homework time?"
- "Why do children demonstrate challenging behavior during homework completion?"
- "Why do children demonstrate undesired behavior when they are bored?"
- "How can you use positive reinforcement to reduce the likelihood your child will engage in behaviors that are negatively reinforcing?"

4.d. *Guide parents to understand the difference between positive reinforcement and bribery.* This is an important distinction, as parents understandably feel uncomfortable if they believe they are bribing their child to behave. Primary distinguishing points: Bribery is generally a *reactive* approach used to get parents out of a bad situation that *reinforces undesirable child behavior*. For example, when your child repeatedly whines for candy in the grocery store, giving in and buying candy is a form of bribery. In contrast, positive reinforcement is a *proactive* and strategic approach that *reinforces desirable behavior*.

> **Pro Tip**
>
> Ignoring is a way to reduce unwanted behaviors without applying punishment. As such, use of ignoring does not factor into computing the 4:1 ratio of reinforcement to punishment.

- "What are your thoughts about the difference between positive reinforcement (or rewards) and bribery?"
- "How can you determine if you are using positive reinforcement or bribery?"

4.e. *Assist parents in understanding the difference between ignoring and punishment.* Ignoring and punishment are both used to reduce the frequency of undesired behavior. The difference is subtle but important. With ignoring, parents make a strategic decision not to reinforce a particular behavior. The baseline condition is neutral (no reinforcement), and parents decide not to introduce reinforcement when a target behavior (e.g., child whining) occurs. With punishment, parents make a strategic decision to remove positive reinforcement. The baseline condition is reinforcing to the child (e.g., parent attention, child engaged in screen time) and parents decide to remove reinforcement as a punishment (e.g., withdraw attention, remove screen time). Ignoring is typically preferable as a consequence for high-frequency behaviors that are not major violations of house rules (e.g., whining, making annoying noises, failing to pay attention).

- "What is the difference between ignoring and punishment?"
- "What is the desired outcome of using ignoring?"
- "When do you use ignoring compared with punishment?"

Session 3: Understanding the Basics of Behavior Management 67

Goal 5—Discuss types of positive reinforcers. (10 minutes)

The session concludes with a brief discussion about different types of positive reinforcement. The purpose of the discussion is to assist parents in generating a menu of reinforcers to deliver to their children in response to desirable behaviors. Another purpose is to help parents understand that reinforcers differ in their developmental appropriateness and that the ultimate goal is for individuals to perform actions for internal or self-reinforcement (e.g., a sense of competence, a sense of doing what is just or good) as opposed to external reinforcement (e.g., obtaining material rewards or praise from others). One of the most powerful strategies parents can use to influence behavior change is the combination of consistently delivering positive reinforcement in response to desired behavior and not giving positive reinforcement (ignoring) in response to undesired behavior.

5.a. *Ask parents to generate examples of positive reinforcers.* The clinician is advised to write responses on a whiteboard or large sheet of paper in accordance with the hierarchy of reinforcement (from highest to lowest: self-reinforcement, attention and praise from others, privileges or tokens to obtain privileges, material objects or tokens to obtain these objects, and food). Distribute the handout *Using Positive Reinforcement* and refer to it to help parents understand the hierarchy of reinforcement types.

- "What sorts of things have you used as positive reinforcement for your child?"
- "What would you consider using as positive reinforcement?"

5.b. *Parents should understand that the effectiveness of reinforcement types can vary across children (i.e., "one size does not fit all").* A child's developmental level is an important factor to consider when attempting to identify effective positive reinforcers. In general, as children advance developmentally, it is recommended to use a higher level of reinforcer. The goal is to get the child to a point at which behavior can be maintained by self-reinforcement. Clinicians should recommend that parents use the highest level of reinforcement in a situation that will be successful in getting their child to perform the targeted behavior. It is also recommended that parents engage their child in developing a range of options for positive reinforcement, as children are often able to identify reinforcers that parents may not consider.

- "What kinds of positive reinforcement have been effective for your child?"
- "How have positive reinforcers you use changed as your child gets older?"
- "What can you do to increase the value of self-reinforcement (i.e., sense of pride, sense of being a good person) for your child?"

Goal 6—Assign homework and identify practice supports for consistent implementation. (5 minutes)

- *Ask parents to complete an A-B-C analysis of two or three problem behaviors over the next week.* They should use the format of the *A-B-C Worksheet* to document their analyses.
- *Parents should create a menu of reinforcers in collaboration with their child.* Encourage parents to include various reinforcement types.

- *Ask parents to practice giving effective instructions.*
- *Encourage parents to continue the Child's Game.*
- *Ask parents to think about their implementation of the A-B-C analysis and Child's Game throughout the week and consider any barriers they face with implementation (provide an example).*
- *Discuss the importance of consistent implementation.* Remind parents that all parents face challenges in using recommended strategies on a frequent and consistent basis.

Session 3 Child Group Agenda

1. Review the group rules and token reinforcement system.
2. Maintain group cohesion.
3. Discuss the role of consequences for behavior.
4. Conclude session.

Materials Needed

- For token reinforcement system—stopwatch/timer (for keeping track of 15-minute intervals) and flip chart
- Name tags
- Deck of playing cards
- Crayons/markers
- Reinforcers that can be used as part of a token reinforcement system
- Snacks for snack break during session

Goal 1—Review the group rules and token reinforcement system.

Escort children into the child therapy room after a brief, joint orientation with their parents. The first goal is to make sure the children are oriented to the group rules that were developed during the initial session and the token reinforcement system.

- Remind children of the group name they agreed on during the initial session.
- Ask children to identify rules that were identified during the initial session.
- Review how the token reinforcement system operates and ask children if they have any questions.
- Review the agenda for the current session and activities.
- Start the first 15-minute interval for the token reinforcement system.

Session 3: Understanding the Basics of Behavior Management 69

Goal 2—Maintain group cohesion.

Building group cohesion was an important part of Sessions 1 and 2. During this third group session, it is important for group leaders to dedicate some time to maintaining good relationships among the group members.

- Ask each child what they liked best about the most recent group session. Each child should be encouraged to talk about at least one thing they enjoyed.
- Ask children to share one thing they enjoy doing outside of school. Praise children for participating. Encourage children to share additional ideas of things they like to do outside of school.

Goal 3—Discuss the role of consequences for behavior.

The goal of this portion of the child group session is to help the children think about the effects of consequences for behavior. The discussion should help children identify consequences they experience in response to their behavior and how consequences have an impact on their behavior.

- Ask children to share some ways they are rewarded for their behavior.
- Engage children in discussion of how getting rewarded for their behavior makes them feel.
- Ask children to share some ways they are punished for their behavior.
- Support children in a discussion about how being punished makes them feel.
- Help children in identifying some ways their behavior changes in response to rewards and punishment.
- Prepare children for the upcoming break, by explaining that all rules still apply, and describing how children will take turns going to the bathroom.

Snack Break

Goal 4—Conclude session.

- Engage children in a card game or art activity, according to their choice, if there is time remaining.
- Announce point totals and allow children to choose prizes. Emphasize positive behaviors displayed by each child. Do not focus on disruptive behaviors. Rather, encourage children to keep up the effort to follow rules throughout the week and at the next session.

CHAPTER 8

FSS Session 4
Preparing for Family–School Collaboration

Session 4 Agenda

1. Review homework assigned last session with a focus on consistent implementation. (20 minutes)
2. Discuss the importance of the teacher–student relationship and family–school collaboration. (10 minutes)
3. Discuss ways to build and sustain partnerships with teachers. (25 minutes)
4. Discuss guidelines for establishing a Daily Report Card. (30 minutes)
5. Assign homework and identify practice supports for consistent implementation. (5 minutes)

Materials Needed

- Handout—*Tips for Building Partnerships with Teachers*
- Handout—*Developing a Daily Report Card*
- Handout—*Sample Daily Report Card (Not Recommended)*
- Handouts—*Sample Daily Report Card (1 and 2)*
- Handouts—*FSS Theory of Change* and *Attention Grid* (both distributed in Session 1)
- Dry-erase markers (to post agenda on whiteboard with time limits for each section if in-person session)

Session Process Reminders

1. Focus on using open-ended questions.
2. Practice reflective listening throughout the session to highlight and build on key points.
3. Validate emotions parents are experiencing related to their parenting.
4. Affirm parents for any effort or movement in the direction of change and implementation of recommended strategies.
5. Support all parents in participating, but avoid putting anyone on the spot.
6. Facilitate the group interacting with each other, rather than just the clinician(s).
7. Keep the group focused on key points and refocus the discussion if it becomes tangential.

Goal 1—Review homework assigned last session with a focus on consistent implementation. (20 minutes)

The families were given several homework assignments at the end of Session 3. It is important to allow time during the start of the current session for parents to share their experiences, receive feedback from other group members and the clinician, and reflect on the importance of homework in supporting consistent implementation of skills.

Collect completed homework assignments and make copies. The purpose of collecting assignments is to promote accountability and encourage consistent implementation. Continue to emphasize the importance of completing homework assignments. Encourage parents to share how they receive support from other caregivers in implementing homework assignments.

1.a. *Ask parents to discuss their experience in completing the A-B-C exercise.* Ask parents to share an example from their A-B-C analysis.
- "What was the exercise like for you?"
- "What behaviors did you target for change?"
- "How did you frame out the target behaviors?"
- "What did you learn about setting your children up for success (identifying antecedents)?"
- "What antecedents helped to set your child up for success? What antecedents did not?"
- "What consequences do you use that maintain undesirable child behaviors?"
- "What consequences do you use that increase the likelihood of appropriate behaviors?"

1.b. *Ask parents to share examples of positive reinforcers they identified since the last session.* Let parents know that you will continue to develop the list so they have a full menu of positive reinforcers.
- "How do you provide positive reinforcement to your child?"
- "What additional positive reinforcement strategies could you use?"

1.c. *Discuss parents' experiences with Child's Game.* Focus on and affirm any efforts parents made to continue making Child's Game part of the daily routine with their child. The clinician should ask parents to identify challenges encountered in implementing Child's Game and strategies used to overcome barriers.

- "How is Child's Game going for you?"
- "How is your child responding?"
- "How can you find time to use this strategy on a regular basis?"

1.d. *Prompt parents to share ways they received support from their partners (or other family members) to complete the homework assignments.* Emphasize the importance of having a strong support system when managing ADHD.

- "How have you involved other caregivers in practicing strategies discussed in this program?"
- "What challenges have you encountered involving other caregivers?"
- "How did you address these challenges?"

Goal 2—Discuss the importance of teacher–student relationship and home–school collaboration. (10 minutes)

The goal of this section is to help parents understand the importance of home–school collaboration to promote their child's success in school. This session is designed to shift the focus of the parents from their home environment to the child's school setting, while continuing to support their efforts to promote behavior change at home.

2.a. *Initiate this section by asking parents to reflect on their own school experiences.* This is designed to help the parents understand their child's perspective about the teacher–student relationship.

- "What was your favorite year of school?"
- "Why was it your favorite?"
- "During your favorite year in school, what difference did the teacher make?"

2.b. *Engage parents in a discussion about the importance of a strong teacher–student relationship.* Strong teacher–student relationships result in positive outcomes for children, including improved school and academic engagement, better academic performance, effective relationships with peers and adults at school, and higher self-esteem.

- "What difference does a strong teacher–student relationship make for your child?"
- "How can this relationship help your child academically, socially, and emotionally?"

2.c. *Ask parents how they can support a positive and effective teacher–student relationship.* The teacher–student relationship is a direct reflection of the family–school relationship. A strong parent–teacher relationship will have a positive effect on the teacher–student relationship.

Pro Tip

This is an important discussion. It is likely to be the first time parents have ever considered how their actions can have an impact on their child's relationship with the teacher, which is critically important for school success.

- "What can you do to strengthen the relationship your children have with their teachers?"
- "How can you work throughout the year to further develop this relationship?"

2.d. *Highlight the importance of building a collaborative family–school relationship.* A strong family–school relationship promotes strong teacher–student relationships, facilitates communication of important information between home and school, and provides the foundation for mutual problem solving.
- "Why is it important to have a strong family–school relationship?"
- "What can you do to establish a strong family–school relationship?"
- "How can you strengthen this relationship during the school year?"

Goal 3—Discuss ways to build and sustain partnerships with teachers. (25 minutes)

In this section the clinician will guide parents in identifying approaches to foster a stronger partnership with their child's teacher or other important adults at school. The discussion should start by acknowledging the efforts parents have already made in establishing collaborative family–school relationships. Following this, parents will share ideas about additional strategies they could use to build effective partnerships. Finally, modeling is recommended to provide parents with examples of ineffective and effective approaches to communication. The clinician should distribute the handout *Tips for Building Partnerships with Teachers*.

3.a. *Ask parents to describe their prior experiences building effective relationships with their child's teachers.* Identify successful strategies the parents are already using.
- "What strategies have you used in the past to communicate effectively with your child's teachers?"
- "What challenges have you faced when trying to build a relationship with your child's teacher?"
- "How have you responded to challenges in a constructive manner?"

3.b. *Encourage parents to share their thoughts about the relationship they have with their child's current teacher.*
- "How would you describe the relationship with your child's current teacher?"
- "If the relationship is going well, how did this happen and what can you do to maintain this?"
- "If the relationship is not going well, what do you think contributed to the current situation?"
- "What ideas do you have about improving the relationship with your child's teacher?"

3.c. *Guide parents in sharing their ideas about building effective partnerships with others, not just teachers.* Some key components might include communicating appreciation of the other, refraining from criticism, acknowledging efforts made by the teacher to be helpful, refraining from giving advice until invited to do so, and following through on commitments to the other person.

- "What are ways to build effective partnerships with others, including teachers?"
- "Thinking about partnerships you have had in the past (including outside of school), what has helped them go well?"

3.d. *Demonstrate approaches to communication via modeling.* We recommend that clinicians initially demonstrate an approach that is NOT RECOMMENDED. One clinician can play the role of the parent and the other the teacher. If there is only one clinician, ask a parent to play the role of the teacher. We suggest that clinicians model a meeting between the parent and teacher that was initiated by the parent due to concerns about the child's behavior or performance. Provide background that the teacher has communicated concerns about the child on several occasions. *Parent role:* Right from the outset, the parent communicates concern about what is happening to the child at school. The parent expresses frustration about hearing complaints and not a plan to improve the situation. In addition, the parent makes suggestions for how the teacher should work with the child. *Teacher role:* The teacher attempts to listen to the parent and reflect concerns expressed by the parent. Over time, the teacher becomes increasingly defensive and frustrated.

Pro Tip

Clinicians may want to consider giving parents an opportunity to practice using recommended strategies for communicating with the teacher. This activity can be somewhat time consuming, so clinicians likely will have to reduce the amount of time they spend discussing other topics.

- "What approaches did the parent use that were not helpful?"
- "How did the teacher respond to the parent?"

3.e. *Next, we recommend that clinicians role-play an approach that is RECOMMENDED. Parent role:* The parent exhibits the following actions: (1) expresses gratitude to the teacher for taking time to meet, (2) asks the teacher to describe concerns about the child and listens nondefensively, (3) acknowledges that the child can be challenging to educate and empathizes with the teacher about how challenging it can be to work with the child, (4) expresses appreciation for the efforts that teacher has made to help the child, and (5) engages the teacher in a discussion about how they can work together to help the child. *Teacher role:* The teacher communicates an interest in helping the child. The teacher provides a brief summary of concerns about the child and expresses appreciation of the parent's willingness to help. The teacher appreciates the support of the parent and engages the parent in a discussion about how they can work together to help the child.

- "What approaches did the parent use that were helpful?"
- "How did the teacher respond? How did the parent's approach set up the teacher's response?"
- "What points do you want to keep in mind when communicating with your child's teacher?"

Goal 4—Discuss guidelines for establishing a Daily Report Card (DRC). (30 minutes)

DRCs provide a way to promote home–school communication and give the child and family specific, frequent feedback about child performance in school. The goals of this portion of the session are to help parents understand the potential value of DRCs, learn the essential components of a DRC, and learn the steps involved in developing a DRC with the child's teacher. Parents should be informed that DRCs are an evidence-based behavioral intervention for children with ADHD. The clinician should distribute the handout *Developing a Daily Report Card*.

4.a. *Initiate the discussion by asking parents if their children already have a DRC or have had one in the past.*
- "Does anyone already use a DRC or have used one in the past?"
- "How does your DRC work?"

4.b. *Share an example of a DRC that is NOT RECOMMENDED.* The following are some potential problems with DRCs. One problem is the use of an "all or nothing" rating system (e.g., happy or sad faces). A dichotomous choice does not acknowledge variations in how children behave, and getting a low rating (e.g., sad face) can be discouraging to the child. The anchor point for the lowest rating should be something like "work harder," instead of "poor." Another problem is stating target behaviors in nonspecific, difficult to observe, negatively worded terms (e.g., "not following rules during math"). The target behavior should indicate what behavior the child should perform more often and not what the child should do less often. A third problem is establishing goals that are too high for the child. A goal should be established so that it is likely the child will achieve it at least 80% of the time. An additional concern is that some DRCs do not allow children to obtain reinforcement for their behavior on a frequent basis (e.g., daily, or several times per day). The clinician should distribute the handout *Daily Report Card—NOT RECOMMENDED*.
- "What concerns do you have with this DRC? Why?"
- "What is a better way to design a DRC?"

4.c. *Provide an example of a DRC that is RECOMMENDED.* Recommended DRCs limit the focus to two to three target behaviors, state the behaviors in specific, observable, and positive terms, provide three or more response choices for teachers, establish realistic goals for children, and provide opportunities for children to receive feedback on a frequent basis. Parents should be encouraged to refer to the handouts *Developing a Daily Report Card*, *Daily Report Card 1*, and *Daily Report Card 2* to guide the discussion about important elements to include in an effective daily report card.
- "What features of this DRC are helpful and likely to be effective? Why?"

4.d. *Guide parents in developing a DRC.* Ask for a volunteer to work with the group to develop a sample DRC for their child. Engage the group in a discussion to develop components of the DRC.
- "What target behaviors would you like to include in your child's DRC?"
- "How can these behaviors be framed to be clear, specific, observable, and positively stated?"

- "What response options would you recommend for evaluating these target behaviors?"
- "How often would you like the teacher to evaluate your child each day?"
- "How would you determine a daily goal for your child?"
- "How do you want to respond when your child achieves the daily goal?"
- "How do you want to respond when your child does not achieve the daily goal?"

4.e. *Engage parents in a discussion about how to successfully implement a DRC for their child.* It is important for parents to involve their children in identifying behaviors to target in a DRC. It is also important for DRCs to be developed in collaboration with teachers. Teachers usually like to start with simple DRCs and build from there. However, some teachers may question the acceptability of using a DRC or question its usefulness for a particular child. If teachers question the usefulness of a DRC, it is often helpful for parents and teachers to identify at least one target behavior to work on together. Teachers can indicate what they will do to help the child with this behavior and parents can state what they will do. Over time, parents and teachers can monitor progress and build the intervention so that it is helpful for the child.

- "How can you involve your child in identifying target behaviors for a DRC?"
- "How would you go about talking to the teacher about starting a DRC?"
- "What can you do to help the DRC intervention get off to a good start?"
- "How do you want to respond if the teacher is not supportive of using a DRC?"

Pro Tip

It is important for DRCs to be developed in the context of a strong collaborative relationship with the teacher. It is usually advisable to start slowly and build the DRC in a way that is acceptable to teachers. We often recommend that daily use of a DRC be included in a student's 504 plan or individualized education program (IEP).

Goal 5—Assign homework and identify practice supports for consistent implementation. (5 minutes)

- *Encourage parents to connect with their child's teacher in the near future.* Encourage parents to rehearse the strategies for building and sustaining a strong parent–teacher partnership.
- *Request that parents work on a draft of a DRC, using the DRC checklist as a guide.* Encourage parents to involve their child in designing the DRC. Inform parents that it is helpful to work on a draft of the DRC, even though the actual DRC developed for their child must include input from the teacher.
- *Inform parents that you or a member of the team will be contacting them by phone during the week to discuss family–school collaboration strategies.* To prepare for this call, ask parents to consider how they could approach a meeting with the school in a way that would be helpful for their child. During the call, discuss with parents strategies for conducting

Pro Tip

Keep in mind that the one of the goals of FSS is to support the empowerment of parents to collaborate effectively with school professionals. Although clinicians can help facilitate family–school connections, it is important to support parents in directly doing this important work with the school.

the family–school meeting and ask if there are any ways in which you could be supportive, including contacting the school directly or participating in a family–school meeting, if feasible. (If you plan to contact the school, be sure to obtain written parent permission to release information to school professionals, and encourage parents to connect with school professionals to give them permission to release information to you.)

- *Encourage parents to continue using Child's Game.*
- *Highlight the importance of consistent implementation.*

Session 4 Child Group Agenda

1. Review the group rules and token reinforcement system.
2. Maintain group cohesion.
3. Discuss the importance of the teacher–student relationship.
4. Conclude session.

Materials Needed

- For token reinforcement system—stopwatch/timer (for keeping track of 15-minute intervals) and flip chart
  - Name tags
  - Deck of playing cards
  - Crayons/markers
  - Reinforcers that can be used as part of a token reinforcement system
  - Snacks for snack break during session

Goal 1—Review the group rules and token reinforcement system.

Escort children into the child therapy room after a brief, joint orientation with their parents. The first goal is to make sure children are oriented to the group rules that were developed during the initial session and the token reinforcement system.

- Remind children of the group name they agreed on during the initial session.
- Ask children to identify rules that were identified during the initial session.
- Review how the token economy operates and ask children if they have any questions.
- Review the agenda for the current session and activities.
- Start the first 15-minute interval for the token reinforcement system.

Goal 2—Maintain group cohesion.

Building group cohesion was an important part of the initial sessions. In subsequent group sessions, it is important for group leaders to dedicate some time to maintaining good relationships among the group members.

- Ask each child what they liked best about the most recent group session. Each child should be encouraged to talk about at least one thing they enjoyed.
- Ask children to share their favorite teacher and a reason why this teacher is their favorite. Praise children for participating. Encourage children to share additional thoughts of what helps them enjoy their teachers.

Goal 3—Discuss the importance of the teacher–student relationship.

The goal of this portion of the child group session is to help children develop an understanding of factors that contribute to positive teacher–student relationships. The discussion should help children think about how positive teacher–student relationships develop and are maintained.

- Ask children to share things they like about teachers.
- Ask children to share their thoughts on what teachers try to do to get along with their students.
- Guide children to reflect on situations that may create difficulty in how students get along with teachers (and teachers get along with students).
- Support children in sharing ideas about how teachers and students can improve their relationship if things are not going well.
- Ask children how their parents can help them get along better with teachers.
- Prepare children for the upcoming break, by explaining that all rules still apply, and describing how children will take turns going to the bathroom.

Snack Break

Goal 4—Conclude session.

- Engage children in a card game or art activity, according to their choice, if there is time remaining.
- Announce point totals and allow children to choose prizes. Emphasize positive behaviors displayed by each child. Do not focus on disruptive behaviors. Rather, encourage children to keep up the effort to follow rules throughout the week and at the next session.

CHAPTER 9

FSS Session 5
Introducing the Token Economy

Session 5 Agenda

1. Review homework assigned last session with a focus on consistent implementation. (25 minutes)
2. Review positive reinforcement and types of reinforcers. (10 minutes)
3. Describe and develop a token economy. (50 minutes)
4. Assign homework and identify practice supports for consistent implementation. (5 minutes)

Materials Needed

- Handout—*Establishing a Token Economy*
- Handout—*Using Positive Reinforcement* (to review; distributed in Session 3)
- Handout—*Homework—Target Behaviors*
- Handout—*Homework—Home Rewards Worksheet*
- Handouts (or posters)—*FSS Theory of Change* and *Attention Grid* (both distributed in Session 1)
- Dry-erase markers (to post agenda on whiteboard with time limits for each section if in-person session)

Session Process Reminders

1. Focus on using open-ended questions.
2. Practice reflective listening throughout the session to highlight and build on key points.
3. Validate emotions parents are experiencing related to their parenting.
4. Affirm parents for any effort or movement in the direction of change and implementation of recommended strategies.
5. Support all parents in participating, but avoid putting anyone on the spot.
6. Facilitate the group interacting with each other, rather than just the clinician(s).
7. Keep the group focused on key points and refocus the discussion if it becomes tangential.

Goal 1—Review homework assigned last session with a focus on consistent implementation. (25 minutes)

The homework assignments given at the end of the previous session focused on strategies to strengthen the family–school relationship and help children perform better in school. It is important to provide enough time at the beginning of this session to allow parents to share their experiences communicating with their child's teacher and developing a DRC.

Collect completed homework assignments and make copies. The purpose of collecting assignments is to increase accountability and encourage consistent implementation. Continue to emphasize the importance of completing homework assignments. Encourage parents to share how they receive support from other caregivers in implementing homework assignments.

1.a. *Discuss with parents their experiences in communicating with their child's teacher.* During the last session, parents were asked to communicate with their child's teacher and attempt to arrange a meeting with the teacher. It is often not feasible for parents to set up a meeting with the teacher in such a short period of time. In addition, some parents may not believe a meeting is necessary. Nonetheless, it is important to encourage parents' efforts to communicate with the teacher and work on strengthening this relationship.

- "What experiences did you have this week communicating with your child's teacher?"
- "What do you appreciate about your child's teacher? Were you able to communicate this to the teacher? If so, how?"
- "How can you continue to work on strengthening the relationship you have with your child's teacher?"
- "If you had the chance to meet with your child's teacher, what went well? What could you have done to make the meeting even more successful?"

1.b. *Encourage parents to share examples of the DRC they developed.* Ask parents to share examples of target behaviors they identified, the scale for evaluating their child's behavior, and rewards selected when goals are achieved. Discuss how they involved their child in developing or adapting the DRC. Clinicians should keep in mind that it may not have been feasible for parents to meet with teachers during the past week to develop a DRC. If they were not able to meet with the teacher, hopefully parents made progress in drafting a DRC with their child. It is important to point out that this is one of the most challenging homework assignments and may take a few weeks to implement.

- "What progress did you make this week in developing or adapting a DRC for your child?"
- "How did you involve your child in this process?"
- "What target behaviors did you select?"
- "What scale did you select to evaluate target behaviors?"
- "What rewards did you identify to reinforce your child for goal attainment?"
- "What are your thoughts about using a DRC with your child?"

1.c. *Discuss parents' experiences with Child's Game.* Focus on and affirm any efforts parents have made to make Child's Game part of the daily routine with their child. Clinicians should work with parents on implementation tools to support frequent use of this critical parenting strategy.

- "What activities are you doing for Child's Game? How is the experience?"
- "What are some of the challenges you are experiencing with Child's Game? How are you trying to address those challenges?"

Goal 2—Review positive reinforcement and types of reinforcers. (10 minutes)

The goal of this section is to briefly review the concept of positive reinforcement and discuss the importance of making positive reinforcement the centerpiece of parenting. It is important for parents to understand that positive parenting is critical for behavior change. In this context, parents need to work on expanding the menu of reinforcers they use to improve target behaviors. Ask parents to refer to the handout *Using Positive Reinforcement* during this discussion.

2.a. *Ask parents to define positive reinforcement.* The purpose of this brief discussion is to promote a deeper understanding of positive reinforcement and why it is so critical for promoting behavior change.

- "We have talked frequently about positive reinforcement. How would you define this concept?"
- "Why is positive reinforcement so critical for promoting your child's success?"

2.b. *Engage parents in a brief discussion about the different types of reinforcers they can use with their child.* It is important for parents to keep working on expanding the menu of reinforcers they use with their child and encouraging children to use self-reinforcement.

- "What methods of positive reinforcement are you using?"
- "How are you using attention and praise to reinforce your child's behavior?"
- "How do you use privileges to reinforce child behavior?"
- "What examples of self-reinforcement (e.g., sense of pride) have you observed in your child? How can you encourage your child's use of self-reinforcement?"

Goal 3—Describe and develop a token economy. (50 minutes)

Token reinforcement is a method of providing salient positive reinforcement to children in a way that is easy and efficient for parents to use. An added advantage is that tokens and points can be provided immediately after desirable behaviors occur. Most parents have some understanding of token reinforcement systems already, although there are often misconceptions about using a token system. During the initial part of this section, it is important for the clinician to help parents understand why most children with ADHD need token systems. Following that, the clinician works with parents to refine their knowledge of this technique and identify ways of applying the strategy at home with their child. The clinician should distribute the handout *Establishing a Token Economy* in the context of this discussion.

> **Pro Tip**
>
> Some parents are skeptical about using token systems, pointing out that their previous efforts to use this approach have failed. In these cases, it is important to affirm parents for their previous efforts and ask if they would be willing to take a fresh look at this strategy.

3.a. *Ask parents to describe their prior experience with token economy systems.* The purpose of this discussion is to introduce the topic of a token economy and build on parents' prior knowledge of this strategy.

- "What is a token economy (also called a token reinforcement system)?"
- "What experiences have you had using a token system?"

3.b. *Help parents understand why children with ADHD often benefit from a token economy.* This discussion should help parents understand that the neurological functioning of children with ADHD generally disposes them to be underresponsive to positive reinforcement. As a result, reinforcers typically provided at home and school (e.g., parental attention and praise) may not be sufficient to promote behavior change. Children with ADHD typically need reinforcers that are more salient. Parents and teachers can increase the salience of rewards by making them concrete (i.e., privileges, material objects) and giving them immediately and frequently. It is usually not feasible to give concrete rewards on a frequent basis. Token systems are a feasible way to give salient rewards on a frequent basis; tokens are easy to administer and can be exchanged in the future for valued, more concrete rewards.

- "Providing attention and praise to children is a powerful strategy, but it may not be sufficient. What other reinforcers have you identified that are effective with your child?"
- "How feasible is it for you to give your child privileges or material rewards on a frequent basis?"
- "How could a token economy approach be helpful to you in your parenting?"

3.c. *Step 1 of building a token economy: Help parents identify reinforcers or rewards they can include in their token system.* Rewards can be differentiated by the frequency with which they can be delivered. Rewards that can be delivered frequently (e.g., parental attention, praise, increments of screen time) are generally less salient than those that can be delivered less frequently (e.g., having a later bedtime, going out for lunch, going on an outing). A useful exercise is to draw four columns on a whiteboard and label each column from left to right with regard to the frequency with which rewards can be given: multiple times per day, once per day, weekend rewards, and long-term rewards. Ask parents to generate a list of rewards they are currently using or could use, and write each reward in the appropriate column. This discussion should help parents identify reward options in each of these categories. In addition, clinicians should provide guidance in assigning token or point values to each of the rewards (i.e., rewards the child will earn frequently are worth fewer points than rewards the child can earn weekly or monthly). Parents should be encouraged to refer to the list of rewards they developed following Session 3 to help guide this discussion.

- "What rewards are you currently giving to your child?"
- "What additional rewards could you use?"
- "How often can you give these rewards to your child?"
  - "Multiple times per day?"
  - "Once a day?"
  - "On the weekends?"
  - "Every few weeks or once a month?"
- "What token or point values would you assign to each of these rewards?"
- "How can you involve your child in identifying rewards?"

3.d. *Step 2 of building a token economy: Guide parents in identifying behavioral goals to target with the token economy.* Parents should be encouraged to focus on a limited number of target behaviors (three or four) when they are setting up a token economy system. Parents are encouraged to identify target behaviors that vary in how difficult they are for children to perform. At least one target behavior should be relatively easy for the child, one should be moderately challenging, and at least one should be challenging to perform. Review the principles of defining target behaviors (framed in a positive manner, specific, observable). Target behaviors should require an active response from the child (that is, they should pass the "dead person's test" as discussed in Session 3). We suggest that you write the target behaviors identified by parents on a whiteboard, and then indicate which behaviors have a low, medium, and high level of difficulty. Finally, guide parents in determining how many points should be given to children for performing a target behavior. Behaviors that are more challenging to perform typically will earn the child more points.

- "What behaviors would you like to target for your child?"
- "How can you frame out these behaviors in positive, specific, and observable terms?"
- "What types of target behaviors do you think will be relatively easy for your child to perform?"
- "What target behaviors do you think will be harder/more challenging?"
- "How can you determine the number of points that should be assigned to each target behavior?"
- "How can you involve your child in identifying target behaviors?"

Pro Tip

The degree of difficulty of target behaviors likely will vary among children. Clinicians can acknowledge this during the discussion. The point of the exercise is to help parents differentiate level of difficulty, which will help them in identifying point values associated with identified target behaviors.

3.e. *Step 3 of building a token economy: Discuss the system for exchanging points/tokens for rewards and a chart for tracking progress.* Parents usually benefit from guidance in establishing a system for their child to exchange points/tokens for rewards. The clinician should emphasize that the process should account for normal household routines and the business of running the house to ensure sustainability. For younger children, it is often helpful to use concrete tangible tokens that are collected in a jar/container. Examples include marbles, cotton balls, poker chips, or pennies. For older children, points can be tallied on paper, whiteboard, or electronic device. It is helpful for the family to create a visual display of the token system that indicates target behaviors, points assigned for each behavior, rewards that can be earned, and the value of each reward. It is critically important to involve children in developing the system in order to gain their cooperation.

- "What would be a good system for keeping track of how many tokens or points your child earns?"
- "What would be a good way to display the behaviors being targeted and the rewards your child can earn?"
- "How can you ensure that the system you use will fit into family routines?"
- "What would be a good time of the day and week for your child to cash in tokens for rewards?"
- "How can you involve your child in developing the system?"

Pro Tip

Although it is a good idea for parents to encourage their children to save points to "cash in" for more valuable rewards, some children may hoard points and rarely cash them in. Hoarding tokens/points may result in the child trading in tokens less often, thus reducing the frequency and immediacy of the child receiving salient rewards. To prevent this from occurring, parents can set a limit on how many points can be carried over each week.

3.f. *Identify potential challenges in implementing a token system and strategies to address the challenges.* Token systems can be challenging for parents to develop and implement. Emphasize the importance of starting with a simple system and developing it over the course of time. Point out that a period of trial and error is needed to work out bugs in the system. Parents often ask about what to do if siblings are also interested in having a token system. Clinicians should encourage parents to adapt the system so it can apply to any sibling who is interested. It is also helpful to point out that DRCs are token systems designed to help children perform well in school. Discuss with parents how points earned on the DRC can be integrated into the home token system.

- "What are your thoughts about developing a token system for your child?"
- "What will be challenging about developing and implementing a token system for your child?"
- "How can you address these anticipated challenges?"
- "How can you adapt your token system so it can be used with siblings?"
- "How can you integrate points earned on the DRC with your home token system?"

Goal 4—Assign homework and identify practice supports for consistent implementation. (5 minutes)

- *Request that parents develop a list of target behaviors with their child and write these on the Homework—Target Behaviors handout.* Ask parents to indicate on the worksheet how many points their child should earn for performing each target behavior.
- *Request that parents expand the reward menu previously developed.* Ask them to assign point values to each reward.
- *Request that parents involve their child in developing the token system.* Parents should be encouraged to complete the *Homework—Home Rewards Worksheet*.
- *Request that parents continue to work on communications with the teacher and efforts to develop a DRC.*
- *Encourage parents to continue implementing Child's Game.*
- *Encourage parents to call you if any questions or concerns arise in the coming week.*

Session 5 Child Group Agenda

1. Review the group rules and token reinforcement system.
2. Maintain group cohesion.
3. Discuss the advantages of a token reinforcement system.
4. Discuss ways to identify reinforcers and promote productive behaviors.
5. Conclude session.

Materials Needed

- For token reinforcement system—stopwatch/timer (for keeping track of 15-minute intervals) and flip chart
- Name tags
- Deck of playing cards
- Crayons/markers
- Paper or whiteboard for Reward Guessing Game
- Reinforcers that can be used as part of a token reinforcement system
- Snacks for snack break during session

Goal 1—Review the group rules and token reinforcement system.

Escort children into the child therapy room after a brief, joint orientation with their parents. The first goal is to make sure the children are oriented to the group rules that were developed during the initial session and the token reinforcement system.

- Remind children of the group name they agreed on during the initial session.
- Ask children to identify rules that were identified during the initial session.
- Review how the token economy operates and ask children if they have any questions.
- Review the agenda for the current session and activities.
- Start the first 15-minute interval for the token reinforcement system.

Goal 2—Maintain group cohesion.

Building group cohesion was an important part of the initial sessions. In subsequent group sessions, it is important for group leaders to dedicate some time to maintaining good relationships among the group members.

- Ask each child what they liked best about the most recent group session. Each child should be encouraged to talk about at least one thing they enjoyed.
- Ask children to share their favorite rewards they receive and a reason why this reward is their favorite. Praise children for participating. Encourage children to share additional thoughts of rewards they appreciate.

Goal 3—Discuss the advantages of a token reinforcement system.

The goal of this portion of the child group session is to help children develop an understanding of how a token economy can support behavioral improvement. The discussion should guide children in reflecting on the use of a token reinforcement system in the group sessions and how such a system can help them at school and home.

- Ask children to identify how the token reinforcement system helps them to have better behavior during the group sessions.
- Ask children their favorite thing about the system.
- Ask children how the system could be improved.
- Play Reward Guessing Game. The goal of this game is to provide children with an opportunity to identify rewards they may like to earn as part of a reward system.
  - Ask each child to think of a reward they would like to earn, write it on a small piece of paper, and then fold it in half so the other children do not see the word.
  - Reward Guessing Game is a *Wheel of Fortune*-style game. The group leader should ask for a volunteer and help the child write on a sheet of paper (or whiteboard if available) blank spaces/squares corresponding with each letter of the reward they identified.
  - Each child in the group takes turns guessing one letter at a time to attempt to spell the word. If a child correctly guesses a letter, they take an additional turn until they make an incorrect guess.

Session 5: Introducing the Token Economy

- The child taking a turn may attempt to guess the entire word(s) during their turn if they are ready to do so.
- After a reward is correctly identified, engage the children in a brief discussion highlighting why this is a desired reward and if other children would like it as well.
- Ask another child to volunteer their reward for the next round.
- Prepare children for the upcoming break, by explaining that all rules still apply, and describing how children will take turns going to the bathroom.

Snack Break

Goal 4—Discuss ways to identify reinforcers and promote productive behaviors.

- Engage children in a role-play activity.
  - Divide the group into two teams.
  - Briefly model a role play of a child talking with their parent(s) about rewards they would like for productive behavior.
  - Ask each team to perform one of the following role plays for the other team.
    - Role play in which children discuss with their parents what rewards they would like to receive for completing their homework
    - Role play in which the child works hard to pay attention to homework and then obtains praise and a reward from their parents for being productive.
  - Find opportunities to praise children's efforts while they are enacting their role plays.
  - Refrain from offering corrective feedback as much as possible.

Goal 5—Conclude session.

- Engage children in a card game or art activity, according to their choice, if there is time remaining.
- Announce point totals and allow children to choose prizes. Emphasize positive behaviors displayed by each child. Do not focus on disruptive behaviors. Rather, encourage children to keep up the effort to follow rules throughout the week and at the next session.

CHAPTER 10

FSS Session 6

Understanding the Function of Behavior and Establishing the Homework Ritual

Session 6 Agenda

1. Review homework assigned last session with a focus on consistent implementation. (30 minutes)
2. Assist parents in analyzing the antecedents and consequences of homework behavior. (25 minutes)
3. Support parents in establishing a homework ritual. (30 minutes)
4. Assign homework and identify practice supports for consistent implementation. (5 minutes)

Materials Needed

- Handout—*Establishing the Homework Ritual*
- Handout—*Homework—Homework A-B-C Worksheet*
- Handout—*Homework—Homework Ritual Worksheet*
- Handouts (or posters)—*FSS Theory of Change* and *Attention Grid* (both distributed in Session 1)
- Dry-erase markers (to post agenda on whiteboard with time limits for each section if in-person session)

Session Process Reminders

1. Focus on using open-ended questions.
2. Practice reflective listening throughout the session to highlight and build on key points.
3. Validate emotions parents are experiencing related to their parenting.
4. Affirm parents for any effort or movement in the direction of change and implementation of recommended strategies.
5. Support all parents in participating, but avoid putting anyone on the spot.
6. Facilitate the group interacting with each other, rather than just the clinician(s).
7. Keep the group focused on key points and refocus the discussion if it becomes tangential.

Goal 1—Review homework assigned last session with a focus on consistent implementation. (30 minutes)

Several homework assignments were provided at the end of Session 5. The primary assignment was for parents to work on initiating a token reinforcement system with their child. Parents were asked to develop a list of target behaviors, assign token/point values to the behaviors, and start using the reinforcement system. In addition, parents were reminded to continue using the Child's Game activity on a daily basis. Given the complexity of starting a token economy, it is important for the clinician to provide sufficient time at the start of the session for parents to share their experiences, ask questions, and receive feedback about their initial implementation efforts.

Collect completed homework assignments and make copies. The purpose of collecting assignments is to increase accountability and encourage consistent implementation. Continue to emphasize the importance of completing homework assignments. Encourage parents to share how they receive support from other caregivers in implementing homework assignments.

1.a. *Ask parents to share examples of target behaviors they identified for the token reinforcement system.* Encourage parents to provide feedback to one another about whether behaviors are framed clearly and in a positive way. Provide support to parents who may experience difficulty identifying appropriate target behaviors.
   - "What behaviors did you choose?"
   - "Why did you select these behaviors?"

1.b. *Encourage parents to share their token reinforcement system.* This is a critical element of the homework review and will likely require much of the time dedicated to this section. Parents should be asked to share their thought process in assigning token/point values to target behaviors, how they provide tokens/points to the child when the target behavior is performed, and the experience of trading tokens/points for rewards. It is important for the clinician to praise and affirm parents' efforts even if modifications are needed.
   - "What are some examples of rewards your child can obtain with their tokens/points?"
   - "How did you determine the number of tokens or points for each target behavior?"

- "What kinds of tokens are you using? How are you keeping track of tokens/points?"
- "How did you figure out how many tokens/points are required to earn a reward?"

1.c. *Support parents who were not able to initiate the token reinforcement system.* It is likely that some of the parents in the group did not start working on their token reinforcement system. There are multiple reasons why this may be the case and identifying and addressing barriers can be useful for participants.
- "What difficulties did you have with starting the token economy?"
- "What did you do to try to overcome the challenge with starting the token economy? What do you plan to try in the coming week?"

1.d. *Discuss parents' experiences in implementing Child's Game.* Focus on and affirm efforts parents have made to continue using this strategy.
- "What activities are you doing for Child's Game?"
- "What are some of the challenges with continuing to use Child's Game each day?"

Pro Tip

Many parents implement Child's Game inconsistently as the program progresses. It is important to keep asking how parents are doing with this and affirming their efforts to sustain use of this foundational strategy.

Goal 2—Assist parents in analyzing the antecedents and consequences of homework behavior. (25 minutes)

Improving children's homework performance is a way to promote family–school collaboration, reduce parent–child conflict, and improve student academic performance. There are many factors that contribute to homework problems and numerous strategies that can improve performance. The A-B-C model is a useful framework for identifying factors contributing to homework problems and strategies for improving homework performance.

2.a. *Initiate this section by reviewing the A-B-C model of behavior.* By this point parents should be very familiar with this model and should be able to define each component of the model.
- "Who can remind us of the A-B-C model of behavior? What do the *A*, *B*, and *C* represent in this model?"

2.b. *Discuss homework behaviors that cause a problem for their children (Behaviors). Select one or two of these behaviors, identify factors that can set children up for each of these homework problems (Antecedents), and identify parent responses and other events that happen after the behavior that might maintain the problem (Consequences).* Clinicians should use a whiteboard to write parents' responses, filling in columns for antecedents, behaviors, and consequences.
- "What is a problematic behavior your child demonstrates when attempting to complete homework?"
- "How does this behavior get in the way of their homework completion?"
- "What is an alternative behavior that would be more likely to support homework completion?"

2.c. *Discuss potential strategies for addressing homework problems.* For the behaviors that were a focus of discussion for 2.b., reframe the problem into a clear target behavior that indicates what children should do (Behavior), identify factors that set children up to succeed for each target behavior (Antecedents), and identify responses to the target behaviors that can increase the likelihood children will respond in an adaptive way (Consequences). Once again, it may be useful to use a whiteboard to write parents' responses, filling in columns for antecedents, behaviors, and consequences. If time permits, it likely will be helpful to identify antecedent and consequent strategies for multiple target homework behaviors.

- "What are some things that make it difficult for your child to complete homework?"
- "If your child had trouble understanding how to do the homework, what are some steps you could take?"
- "What are some ways that you try to make it more likely that your child will complete their homework?"
- "What are some things that happen after your child displays behavior that interferes with homework completion?"
- "What are ways that your child's problematic behavior during homework completion may be rewarding?"

Goal 3—Support parents in establishing a homework ritual. (30 minutes)

This section focuses on helping parents identify antecedent strategies to set their children up for homework success. Specifically, the parents are guided in examining the "where," "when," and "what" of homework completion, also referred to as the "homework ritual." A consistent homework ritual is important to address the poor organizational skills and task avoidance behavior of children with ADHD.

3.a. *Introduce the three W's of homework completion: Where, When, and What. Discuss the "where" of homework.* "Where" refers to the location in which children do their homework. The family should try to select a location that minimizes distractions, enables parents to supervise homework without being overly intrusive, and enables parents to offer praise frequently when indicated. Parents should be encouraged to refer to the handout *Establishing the Homework Ritual*.

- "Where does your child currently complete homework?"
- "What are some positive things about that location? What are some challenges presented by doing homework in that location?"
- "What may be better places for your child to complete their homework?"
- "How can you modify the current location to better support successful homework completion?"

3.b. *Discuss the "when" of homework.* "When" refers to the time of day children do their homework. The family should try to select a time that capitalizes on when the child is likely to be most productive and the parent can supervise effectively.

- "When does your child currently complete homework?"
- "How well does this work?"
- "What factors do you need to think about when deciding when your child should complete homework?"

Pro Tip

If the child is prescribed medication, the homework routine should take into consideration times of the day when medication is still effective.

3.c. *Discuss the "what" of homework completion.* "What" refers to knowing what work has been assigned and having the necessary materials readily available to do the work. Knowing what to do often requires effective family–school communication and teaching children organization skills. Parents should keep in mind that the primary purpose of homework is to practice and master skills taught in school.

- "What materials does your child need to start and stick with completing their homework?"
- "What system is in place to ensure you and your child know what assignments have been given for homework?"
- "How can you collaborate with your child's teacher to ensure your child is prepared to do homework assignments?"
- "What help does your child need to make sure they have the books, worksheets, technology devices, and all other materials needed to start and complete homework?"
- "How can you help your child make sure they have all materials (e.g., pencils/pens, worksheets, notebooks, books) for homework organized and available?"

Pro Tip

It is helpful for parents to collaborate with teachers to develop homework-tracking systems and checklists to ensure children know what to do for homework and have all required materials.

Goal 4—Assign homework and identify practice supports for consistent implementation. (5 minutes)

- *Request that parents complete the Homework A-B-C Worksheet for two or three target homework behaviors (what they want their child to do more often).*
- *Encourage parents to collaborate with their child in establishing their homework ritual and summarize components of the routine on the Homework Ritual Worksheet.*
- *Encourage parents to continue Child's Game.*
- *Ask parents to continue their efforts to implement a token reinforcement system.* Emphasize that the system does not need to be perfect to get started.

Session 6: The Function of Behavior and the Homework Ritual 93

- *Encourage parents to call you if any questions or concerns arise in the coming week.* Emphasize the importance of implementing the homework assignment.
- *Ask parents to think about their implementation of the homework ritual and identify any barriers they encounter in implementing these homework assignments and strategies for reducing these barriers.*

Session 6 Child Group Agenda

1. Review the group rules and token reinforcement system.
2. Maintain group cohesion.
3. Discuss homework successes and problems.
4. Help children improve homework routines and identify potential reinforcers.
5. Conclude session.

Materials Needed

- For token reinforcement system—stopwatch/timer (for keeping track of 15-minute intervals) and flip chart
- Name tags
- Deck of playing cards
- Crayons/markers
- Cards for Concentration Game
- Reinforcers that can be used as part of a token reinforcement system
- Snacks for snack break during session

Goal 1—Review the group rules and token reinforcement system.

Escort children into the child therapy room after a brief, joint orientation with their parents. The first goal is to make sure children are oriented to the group rules that were developed during the initial session and the token reinforcement system.

- Remind children of the group name they agreed on during the initial session.
- Ask children to identify rules that were identified during the initial session.
- Review how the token economy operates and ask children if they have any questions.
- Review the agenda for the current session and activities.
- Start the first 15-minute interval for the token reinforcement system.

Goal 2—Maintain group cohesion.

Building group cohesion was an important part of the initial sessions. In subsequent group sessions, it is important for group leaders to dedicate some time to maintaining good relationships among the group members.

- Ask each child what they liked best about the most recent group session. Each child should be encouraged to talk about at least one thing they enjoyed.
- Ask children to share a time when they were successful with schoolwork or on a test and the thoughts and feelings they experienced. Praise children for participating. Encourage children to share additional experiences and thoughts of school success.

Goal 3—Discuss homework successes and problems.

The goal of this portion of the child group session is to support children in sharing their thoughts and feelings about homework. We suggest using a Concentration Game to help children feel comfortable sharing their thoughts and feelings.

- Prior to the session, the group leader should create a set of Concentration Game cards. One side of each card should have a question or statement written on it about homework (e.g., Name one thing that is hard about homework). The cards should be created in pairs, with each pair including the same question/statement. Other pairs of cards should be created with pictures (such as animals, smiling faces, common objects). Cards can be the size of one-half of a 3 × 5 index card.
- Have children sit in a circle while the group leader places the cards face down in a random order to form a square grid.
- One by one, each child is instructed to choose two cards that are identical to each other (i.e., have the same question or same picture). The child gets a point if they either adequately answer a question or pick a pair of pictures. All children are encouraged to answer the question.

Snack Break

Goal 4—Help children improve homework routines and identify potential reinforcers.

Introduce the Fabulous Four Game. This game provides an opportunity for children to describe their homework routines, including **where**, **when**, **what**, and with **whom** they complete their homework

- Divide the group into two teams.
- Each team needs to provide at least two appropriate answers to each question asked (e.g., "Name places **where** it is good to do your homework," "Name bad places to do your homework," "Name times of the day **when** it is good to do your homework," "Name **what**

materials you need to have with you when you do your homework," and "Describe **who** can help you with homework and how").

- Teams will take turns being the first to answer questions.
- Each team has 2 minutes to answer each question.
- Each team receives 1 point for each question they answer appropriately.
- Use a colorful visual aid to record points earned.

Goal 5—Conclude session.

- Engage children in a card game or art activity, according to their choice, if there is time remaining.
- Announce point totals and allow children to choose prizes. Emphasize positive behaviors displayed by each child. Do not focus on disruptive behaviors. Rather, encourage children to keep up the effort to follow rules throughout the week and at the next session.

CHAPTER 11

FSS Session 7
Managing Time and Goal Setting

Session 7 Agenda

1. Review homework assigned last session with a focus on consistent implementation. (25 minutes)
2. Assist parents in establishing appropriate time limits for their child to do homework. (20 minutes)
3. Guide parents in helping their children develop time management and goal-setting skills using modeling, role play, and guided practice. (40 minutes)
4. Assign homework and identify practice supports for consistent implementation. (5 minutes)

Materials Needed

- Handout—*Managing Time and Goal Setting*
- Handout—*Goal-Setting Tool* (provide copies for each parent)
- Handouts (or posters)—*FSS Theory of Change* and *Attention Grid* (both distributed in Session 1)
- Dry-erase markers (to post agenda on whiteboard with time limits for each section if in-person session)

Session Process Reminders

1. Focus on using open-ended questions.
2. Practice reflective listening throughout the session to highlight and build on key points.
3. Validate emotions parents are experiencing related to their parenting.
4. Affirm parents for any effort or movement in the direction of change and implementation of recommended strategies.
5. Support all parents in participating, but avoid putting anyone on the spot.
6. Facilitate the group interacting with each other, rather than just the clinician(s).
7. Keep the group focused on key points and refocus the discussion if it becomes tangential.

Goal 1—Review homework assigned last session with a focus on consistent implementation. (25 minutes)

At the conclusion of Session 6, parents were asked to complete homework assignments that primarily focused on the antecedents of homework completion. Parents were encouraged to complete A-B-C analyses of problematic homework behaviors and establish the components of their homework ritual. The group leader should provide time for parents to share their experiences with the A-B-C behavioral analysis and homework ritual. Additionally, parents should be given time to share about their implementation of the token reinforcement system and continuing use of Child's Game.

Collect completed homework assignments and make copies. The purpose of collecting assignments is to increase accountability and encourage consistent implementation. Continue to emphasize the importance of completing homework assignments. Encourage parents to share how they receive support from other caregivers in implementing homework assignments.

1.a. *Ask parents to share what they learned from completing the Homework A-B-C Worksheet.* Encourage parents to share target behaviors identified, changes in their homework routine to set their children up for homework success, and consequences being used to increase the likelihood of productive homework behaviors.

- "What did you learn from completing the A-B-C analysis about homework behavior?"
- "What are the components of your homework ritual?"
- "What are you observing since making changes in your homework ritual?"

1.b. *Ask parents about their experiences using the token reinforcement system.* At this point, it is expected that families will have made some effort to initiate a token reinforcement system, although it is possible one or more families have not done so yet. Provide parents an opportunity to share their experiences with implementation and affirm any successes they have had, acknowledging the challenges of doing so.

Pro Tip

Emphasize the importance of progress over perfection in implementing the token economy system.

- "What has been your experience using a token system?"
- "What are you observing about your child's behavior since starting the token economy?"
- "What challenges are you running into with the token system?"

1.c. *Discuss parents' experiences in implementing Child's Game.* Focus on and affirm efforts parents have made to continue using this strategy.
- "What activities are you doing for Child's Game?"
- "What are some of the challenges with continuing to use the Child's Game each day?"

Goal 2—Assist parents in establishing appropriate time limits for their child to do homework. (20 minutes)

When provided with a task, children with ADHD often waste time and fail to persist. Homework can be particularly frustrating given the level of effort necessary and the length of time required. It is important for parents to establish appropriate time limits for homework.

2.a. *Help parents understand the rationale for having a time limit for homework.* It is important for parents to understand "the law of diminishing returns" with homework, that is, working on homework beyond a reasonable time limit often is self-defeating and may increase the problems associated with homework completion. A general rule of thumb for time dedicated to homework completion is approximately 10 minutes per grade level; therefore, asking a second-grade child to spend an hour doing homework, for example, will usually create additional homework problems. However, the child's teacher is usually the best source for guidance about setting an appropriate time limit for homework.
- "How much time is your child spending doing homework?"
- "How productive is your child when doing homework?"
- "What is a reasonable amount of time for your child to spend doing homework?"

2.b. *Assist parents in working through concerns about ending homework when the time limit has expired if assignments are not yet complete.* Parents often express concerns about the consequences of ending homework before all work is completed and done accurately. Parents usually benefit by engaging in a discussion about the benefits and costs of having children work until all work is done accurately. It is also helpful for parents to think through the potential consequences of leaving some work incomplete and inaccurate when the time limit for homework has been reached.
- "What happens when your child works on homework beyond a reasonable time limit? What are the benefits and costs?"
- "What would happen if you allowed your child to do homework only for a set period of time?"
- "How concerned would you be if your child did not complete all homework in a reasonable period of time?"

2.c. *Help parents understand the critical importance of collaborating with teachers to establish time limits for homework and work through challenges in completing homework.* We have found that a high percentage of teachers are very supportive of families who experience challenges with homework completion. Teachers generally are not aware of children's homework challenges unless parents reach out to share this information. Teachers do not want to exacerbate parent–child conflict and child avoidance of schoolwork by having negative homework experiences. It is important to engage parents in a discussion about how they can work with teachers to identify realistic time limits for homework, identify strategies parents can use when children do not complete all their work (e.g., parent sends a note to teacher), and address other problems that can arise with homework (e.g., child and parent do not know what homework has been assigned; child does not have the materials needed to do homework; homework assignment may be too challenging for the child).

- "How could your child's teacher be helpful in identifying realistic time limits for homework and a strategy about what to do when your child does not complete all homework assigned?"
- "How could your child's teacher be helpful in addressing other homework challenges you are facing?"
- "What challenges do you foresee about having this discussion and how could you address these challenges?"

Goal 3—Guide parents in helping their children develop time management and goal-setting skills using modeling, role play, and guided practice. (40 minutes)

Parents usually need substantial guidance in working with their children during homework time. This part of the session is designed to educate parents about a strategy to help with time management and goal setting during homework. It is important to help parents understand that their role in supporting homework is to serve as a coach, rather than attempting to teach the child content that is difficult for the child. The parent can provide brief tutoring to the child on an occasional basis. However, if the child frequently has difficulty understanding the material assigned for homework, it is important for the parent to inform the child's teacher and discuss ways to give the child more academic support. The specific steps of the strategy are outlined in the handouts *Managing Time and Goal Setting* and *Goal-Setting Tool*. Step-by-step directions are outlined below to guide the clinician in modeling and role play during this portion of the session. When FSS is co-led by clinicians or a clinician with trainees, one of the group leaders can take the role of parent and the other can be the child. If the program is being led by a single clinician, the clinician can enlist one of the parents to play the role of child.

3.a. *Demonstrate the use of time management and goal-setting procedures.* The clinician demonstrates the strategy in the context of a role play. Subsequently, the clinician leads the parents in a discussion about the strategy and what parents think about it.

1. Schools use a range of ways to communicate homework assignments (e.g., assignment book, teacher's website, online "parent portal"). Parents should use the method provided by the child's school to review the homework assigned for that day. Based on the work assigned, segment homework into manageable units of time. Each unit should be relatively brief and will vary depending on the grade level of the child and the child's ability to work independently. A general guideline is for the length of time (number of minutes) of a homework unit to be about three times the grade level of the child. For example, a third grader might be expected to work for 9-minute units. Homework assignments can be "chunked" into tasks that should take one unit to complete. In our third-grade example, the homework would be broken up into 9-minute chunks. Longer assignments can be divided into multiple units to make them more manageable for students to complete independently. In other words, if an assignment is likely to take the child longer than one unit to complete, that assignment could be split into two or more units.

2. The parent and child select a unit of work to start homework. It is often advisable to start with an assignment preferred by the child and one that can be accomplished without much difficulty in order to build some momentum. For the purpose of role play, we often use a worksheet of 20 math problems tailored for a second grader. We demonstrate that the child may be overwhelmed in working on so many problems at once, so we divide the page in half, create two subunits, and ask the child to work on one subunit at a time.

3. Parent and child negotiate goals for the first subunit of homework. Goals for work completion, work accuracy, and time to complete work are entered on the *Goal-Setting Tool* handout. The parent includes the child in the process of establishing goals. Demonstrate for parents where this information is entered on the *Goal-Setting Tool* handout.

> **Pro Tip**
>
> Children often overestimate goals for their homework performance. It is important for parents to guide children in setting realistic goals for work completion and accuracy so children succeed at least 80% of the time.

4. The parent reviews the directions for the selected assignment with the child to make sure the child understands what is required. In addition, the parent can ask the child to do the first problem with the parent present to ensure understanding.

5. Have the child start working on the first unit of work. Parents should use a countdown timer (e.g., kitchen timer, timer on a cell phone) to ensure adherence to the time limit established for a unit of work. For the purpose of role play, we often set the timer for 2–3 minutes but remind parents that a suggested time limit is approximately three times the child's grade level.

6. While the child in the role play is working on the first unit, the parent is busy doing something else but observing the child carefully. The parent should give frequent praise for attention and effort and ignore inattention and unproductive behavior. If inattention persists for more than about 10 seconds, the parent provides correction briefly by prompting the child to get back to work. Remember, the parent is a coach, not a teacher; therefore, the parent should avoid a tendency to hover over the child in order to promote independence. If the child asks for help, the parent tells the child to do their best until the time period is over.

7. At the end of the work period, the next step is to evaluate the child's performance. The parent and child review the work completed during the time period. Parents assist the child

in determining the number of items completed and the number of items that are correct. This information is entered by the child in Step 2 of the *Goal-Setting Tool*.

8. The parents and child evaluate if the completion and accuracy goals were met during the work period. This is completed at Step 3 on the *Goal-Setting Tool*. The child receives ratings and points for exceeding the goal and meeting the goal.

9. If items have not been completed or are not accurate, the parent can provide the correct answer. We strongly recommend that parents refrain from asking children to go back and correct their work so the child can complete all assigned homework tasks in a reasonable period of time.

10. The parent and child then move on to the next unit of work and start the goal-setting procedure again.

3.b. *Engage parents in a discussion of their thoughts about the goal-setting strategy.* Parents usually have many reactions, because the strategy is likely to be different from their current approach. In particular, parents often have questions about the recommendation for the child not to go back and complete missing or incorrect items after each unit of work is finished. It is usually helpful to remind parents of the goal of homework, which is to help children master academic skills and develop good work habits (including strategies for managing time, setting goals, and evaluating performance). Homework can be counterproductive if it increases frustration and avoidance of academic work and contributes to conflict in the parent–child relationship.

> **Pro Tip**
>
> Some parents continue to be skeptical about using the goal-setting strategy even after discussion. Use motivational interviewing strategies and roll with resistance and skepticism.

- "What are your initial thoughts about the homework goal-setting strategy?"
- "What questions do you have about using this approach with your child?"
- "How do you feel about moving on to the next unit of homework if your child has not completed the previous unit?"

3.c. *Organize the parents in the group into dyads to engage in practice with the homework goal-setting strategy.* If there are two parents from the same family, they can form a dyad. Each parent in the dyad will have a chance to practice being in the parent role and the child role. The clinician should provide parents fresh worksheets to use during practice sessions. During the practice period, the clinician should spend some time with parents in each dyad providing feedback with an emphasis on giving praise for effective use of the goal-setting strategy. Afterward, the clinician should engage parents in another brief discussion of the strategy.

- "What additional thoughts do you have about the goal-setting strategy?"
- "What challenges do you think you will have implementing the strategy and how can you address these?"
- "How could you apply this strategy to tasks in addition to homework?"
- "How can you integrate the homework goal-setting strategy with your token reinforcement system?"

Goal 4—Assign homework and identify practice supports for consistent implementation. (5 minutes)

- *Encourage parents to implement the goal-setting strategy during the week.* We typically recommend that parents implement the strategy two to three times during the coming week. The clinician should provide parents with copies of the goal-setting tool and make this available to them electronically.
- *Encourage parents to communicate with the child's teacher about homework concerns (such as homework is taking excessive time to complete, assignments appear overly challenging for the child's skill level).* If the parents have concerns about how the teacher will react if they use the goal-setting strategy and the child does not complete all homework assigned, they should collaborate with the teacher to identify a strategy to use.
- *Inform parents that a member of the team will be contacting them during the week to discuss family–school collaboration strategies regarding homework.* To prepare for this call, ask parents to identify points they want to share with their child's teacher (e.g., how long child is spending doing homework; how challenging some of the work is; confusion about what homework is being assigned for a particular subject). In addition, it is usually important for parents to discuss how they are supporting their child with homework (e.g., using the goal-setting strategy). Parents can ask the teacher what they should do if all homework items are not completed and/or not completed accurately. During this phone call, the role of the clinician is to provide assistance to parents in developing an agenda for the family–school meeting and considering ways to communicate effectively with the teacher.
- *Encourage parents to continue Child's Game.*
- *Encourage parents to call you if any questions or concerns arise in the coming week.*
- *Discuss the importance of consistent implementation.* Ask parents to think about their implementation of the homework ritual and goal-setting strategy as well as any barriers they face with implementation (provide an example).

Session 7 Child Group Agenda

1. Review the group rules and token reinforcement system.
2. Maintain group cohesion.
3. Provide children with an overview of the homework goal-setting strategy.
4. Engage children in role-play practice of homework goal setting.
5. Conclude session.

Materials Needed

- For token reinforcement system—stopwatch/timer (for keeping track of 15-minute intervals) and flip chart
- Name tags

- Deck of playing cards
- Crayons/markers
- Sample of a homework sheet of math problems (second- or third-grade level)
- Reinforcers that can be used as part of a token reinforcement system
- Snacks for snack break during session

Goal 1—Review the group rules and token reinforcement system.

Escort children into the child therapy room after a brief, joint orientation with their parents. The first goal is to make sure children are oriented to the group rules that were developed during the initial session and the token reinforcement system.

- Remind children of the group name they agreed on during the initial session.
- Ask children to identify rules that were identified during the initial session.
- Review how the token economy operates and ask children if they have any questions.
- Review the agenda for the current session and activities.
- Start the first 15-minute interval for the token reinforcement system.

Goal 2—Maintain group cohesion.

Building group cohesion was an important part of the initial sessions. In subsequent group sessions, it is important for group leaders to dedicate some time to maintaining good relationships among the group members.

- Ask each child what they liked best about the most recent group session. Each child should be encouraged to talk about at least one thing they enjoyed.
- Ask children to share their favorite activities to do after they finish homework and a reason why this is their favorite activity. Praise children for participating. Encourage children to share additional favorite activities after schoolwork is completed.

Goal 3—Provide children with an overview of the homework goal-setting strategy.

The primary goal of the child group session is to orient children to the homework goal-setting strategy their parents are learning. The discussion should help children understand the goal-setting approach to completing homework and how this may differ from their current approach.

- Ask children to identify how they currently approach completing homework assignments.
- Ask children to share ideas about how homework completion could be improved.

- Introduce homework goal setting to the children. Emphasize that homework goal setting is a way to help children get more work done in less time. Here are some questions to discuss with the children.
  - "What is hard about completing your homework?"
  - "Some assignments take a long time to complete. How can you break a long assignment into chunks?"
  - "How long can you work on an assignment before you get bored?"
  - "Some assignments are hard to do. It may not be possible to do all the homework problems correctly. What is a good goal for you with math homework? What about reading/language arts? Science?"
  - "Let's say your goal for math homework is to get 8 of 10 problems correct. After working on your math homework, you and your parent figure out that you have completed 9 of 10 problems correctly. What would be a good reward for meeting your goal?"
- Prepare children for the upcoming break, by explaining that all rules still apply, and describing how children will take turns going to the bathroom.

Snack Break

Goal 4—Engage children in role-play practice of homework goal setting.

- Ask one of the children to volunteer to participate in a role play with one of the group leaders.
- Present the child participating in the role play with a sheet of math problems (as a model homework assignment).
- Guide the child through the initiation of the goal-setting strategy, following the guidance on the *Goal-Setting Tool* handout. The group leader should emphasize each step of the goal-setting strategy for the rest of the children.
- Following this initial role play, the group leader should engage in a role play with another volunteer.
- Provide children with an opportunity to ask questions after each role play.
- Find opportunities to praise children's efforts while they are enacting their role plays.

Goal 5—Conclude session.

- Engage children in a card game or art activity, according to their choice, if there is time remaining.
- Announce point totals and allow children to choose prizes. Emphasize positive behaviors displayed by each child. Do not focus on disruptive behaviors. Rather, encourage the children to keep up the effort to follow rules throughout the week and at the next session.

CHAPTER 12

FSS Session 8
Using Punishment Successfully

Session 8 Agenda

1. Review homework assigned at last session with a focus on consistent implementation. (25 minutes)
2. Provide an overview of the purpose, benefits, and potential adverse effects of punishment. (15 minutes)
3. Discuss strategies for implementing punishment successfully. (45 minutes)
4. Assign homework and identify practice supports for consistent implementation. (5 minutes)

Materials Needed

- Handout—*Using Punishment Successfully*
- Handout—*Punishment Discussion Questions*
- Homework—*Using Punishment Strategically*
- Handouts (or posters)—*FSS Theory of Change* and *Attention Grid* (both distributed in Session 1)
- Dry-erase markers (to post agenda on whiteboard with time limits for each section if in-person session)

Session Process Reminders

1. Focus on using open-ended questions.
2. Practice reflective listening throughout the session to highlight and build on key points.

3. Validate emotions parents are experiencing related to their parenting.
4. Affirm parents for any effort or movement in the direction of change and implementation of recommended strategies.
5. Support all parents in participating, but avoid putting anyone on the spot.
6. Facilitate the group interacting with each other, rather than just the clinician(s).
7. Keep the group focused on key points and refocus the discussion if it becomes tangential.

Goal 1—Review homework assigned last session, with a focus on consistent implementation. (25 minutes)

At the conclusion of Session 7, parents were asked to practice using the time management and goal-setting strategy with their child. In addition, they were encouraged to speak with their child's teacher about time limits for homework and concerns about child completion of homework. The clinician should encourage parents to share their experiences using the goal-setting strategy. In addition, the clinician should ask parents to discuss any communication they had with their child's teacher about homework, as well as check in about parents' experiences continuing to use Child's Game.

Collect completed homework assignments and make copies. Continue to emphasize the importance of completing homework assignments. Encourage parents to share how they receive support from other caregivers in implementing homework assignments.

1.a. *Ask parents to share their experiences using the homework goal-setting tool.* Most of the time during homework review should be dedicated to giving parents opportunities to share their experiences using this strategy. This can be a challenging strategy for families at first, so affirmation of implementation efforts is important. Emphasize that it is typical for parents and children to need time and practice to feel comfortable using this approach.

- "What was it like for you using the homework goal-setting strategy?"
- "In what ways has this strategy been helpful for your child?"
- "What challenges have you encountered using this approach?"
- "How does your child feel about this approach?"

1.b. *Ask parents if they had the chance to communicate with their child's teacher about homework time limits and other challenges.* Emphasize that communication with teachers can take many forms, including notes on homework assignments, brief emails, and text messages (if appropriate), in addition to phone calls, virtual meetings, and in-person discussions. In addition, remind parents about the importance of catching teachers being helpful (e.g., trying different approaches with their child), spending extra time with their child, and being responsive to parents. This also is a good time to check in with parents about progress in using the daily report card.

- "Did you communicate with your child's teacher recently? How did it go?"
- "How was the teacher helpful to you in addressing your child's homework challenges?"
- "How are you doing implementing a daily report card with your child?"

Session 8: Using Punishment Successfully 107

- "How did you let the teacher know you appreciate their help?"
- "What could you do in the next week or so to communicate with the teacher?"

1.c. *Discuss parents' experiences in implementing Child's Game.* Focus on and affirm efforts parents have made to continue using this strategy.

- "What activities are you doing for Child's Game?"
- "What are some of the challenges with continuing to use Child's Game each day?"

Goal 2—Provide an overview of the purpose, benefits, and potential adverse effects of punishment. (15 minutes)

Up to this point in the program, the primary focus has been on using positive reinforcement as a consequence-based strategy to increase the frequency of targeted behaviors. Punishment is another consequence that can be highly effective in changing child behavior, if used strategically. Most parents use punishment too frequently and struggle to maintain a 4:1 ratio of positive and neutral feedback to punitive responses. This section is designed to introduce punishment, discuss its purpose, consider the benefits of this strategy when used appropriately, and identify potential adverse effects when used inappropriately. The clinician should distribute the handout *Using Punishment Successfully*.

2.a. *Start off by discussing the purpose of punishment.* Punishment is a consequence-based strategy designed to reduce the frequency of a targeted behavior. When punishment is administered effectively, and used in combination with positive reinforcement, it increases the likelihood that an alternative, desirable behavior will occur. As such, the purpose of punishment is to support teaching children how to behave in a particular situation. Sometimes punishment may have short-term emotional benefits for the parent by enabling them to express frustration or anger, but punishment is not designed to make a parent feel better in the moment or to exact retribution on the child. On the contrary, it is designed to be beneficial for the child.

- "What is punishment?"
- "What is the purpose of punishment?"
- "How can you tell if punishment is being effective?"

2.b. *Discuss the benefits and potential adverse effects of punishment.* When punishment is administered effectively, children learn that in a particular situation one set of behaviors is unacceptable and another set of behaviors is acceptable. When punishment is overused or delivered in a manner that is ineffective, there can be adverse effects, such as an increase in child oppositional and aggressive behaviors, an erosion of the parent–child relationship, and a reduction in child self-esteem.

- "What are the potential benefits of punishment when delivered effectively?"
- "What are potential harmful effects of punishment when delivered too frequently or harshly?"
- "What alternatives to punishment can you use to make sure you are not overusing this approach?"

2.c. *Discuss the difference between punishment and ignoring.* As a rule, parents punish their children too frequently and underuse the strategy of ignoring. As indicated, punishment is the delivery of a consequence after an undesirable behavior in order to reduce the frequency of the target behavior. Ignoring is the strategic decision to withhold adult attention, praise, and other types of positive reinforcement in response to an undesired target behavior. Based on the principle of extinction, persistent use of ignoring will result in a target behavior occurring less frequently. Ignoring can be difficult for parents to deliver, because initial use of the strategy will result in the child's behavior getting worse ("extinction burst"). However, persistent use of the strategy will lead to expected change. Ignoring is the preferred strategy to use with target behaviors that occur frequently and are not major violations of family rules (e.g., whining, making noises, being intrusive). Punishment is the preferred strategy for behaviors that occur less frequently and are major violations of family rules (e.g., hitting, throwing objects, stealing, harming someone emotionally). When combined with consistent positive reinforcement in response to more desirable behavior, the use of punishment and ignoring can result in increased rates of alternative, more adaptable behavior. To help parents effectively use punishment versus ignoring, part of this discussion should focus on identifying major "house rules" that when violated will result in punishment.

- "What is ignoring? How is ignoring different from punishment?"
- "What are examples of behaviors that should be targets of ignoring?"
- "What are examples of behaviors that should be targets of punishment?"
- "What are major rules in your family that should be the targets of punishment?"
- "What challenges do you experience in ignoring your child? How can you work through these challenges?"

Goal 3—Discuss strategies for implementing punishment successfully. (45 minutes)

The rest of the session is devoted to a discussion of specific strategies for implementing punishment and methods for delivering punishment in a manner that will be effective. Most parents have good ideas about effective ways to use punishment, so the discussions are designed to elicit the wisdom parents have and give them opportunities to share their wisdom with each other. Distribute the handout *Punishment Discussion Questions* to help guide group discussion related to effectively using punishment.

3.a. *Discuss different ways to implement punishment effectively.* Inform parents that there are essentially two types of punishment. One type is the removal of positive reinforcement (sometimes referred to as *negative punishment* because something is removed to reduce the frequency of the behavior). Ask parents to identify examples, which could

Pro Tip

Some clinicians use the terms *negative punishment* and *positive punishment* to refer to the two types of punishment. Although this distinction is useful for professionals and trainees, we have found that it can confuse parents. As such, we do not recommend using these terms when communicating with parents in FSS.

include withdrawing parental attention, removing access to privileges, and time out from opportunities to obtain any positive reinforcement, referred to simply as *time out*. The other type is the application of aversive consequences (sometimes referred to as *positive punishment* because something is added or given to reduce the frequency of the behavior). Once again, ask parents to identify examples of this type of punishment, such as requiring a child to do something helpful for a sibling (e.g., doing a sibling's chores) as a consequence for hitting the sibling. By far the most commonly used aversive consequence is verbal correction. This is a good time to point out that effective verbal correction informs the child clearly and briefly what to do instead of what not to do (e.g., "you need to get back to work," instead of "stop looking out the window"). This is also a good time to point out that we never recommend the use of physical punishment, because of the risk of harmful side effects, including child abuse.

- "What punishment strategies do you use that involve taking away positive reinforcement? Are there other ways you could do this?"
- "How can you use aversive consequences as a punishment strategy for your child?"
- "How often do you give your child verbal correction?"

Pro Tip

Parents are often surprised to learn that verbal correction is a form of punishment. It is important for parents to understand this point in order to adhere to the 4:1 principle (giving at least four times more positive and neutral feedback as opposed to corrective feedback).

- "What alternative approaches could you use to reduce the number of times you give your child verbal correction?"
- "What are effective ways to give verbal correction?"
- "What are the problems with using physical punishment with your child?"

3.b. *Discuss principles for delivering punishment effectively.* Point out important principles of behavior change: consistency, immediacy, specificity (targeting specific behaviors), saliency (using consequences that are meaningful to the child), and 4:1, which we often refer to as the *CISS-4 principles*. When delivering punishment, it is important to be firm, clear, and under emotional control: in other words, to mean what you say. Another principle to keep in mind is that punishment needs to be relatively brief. Once again, the purpose of punishment is to educate the child and not to exact retribution. Lengthy punishments can be counterproductive in that they can lead to resentment. In addition, if a child is being punished for an extended period (e.g., loss of screen time for an entire evening), the parent forfeits the ability to use this punishment if another situation requiring punishment arises during that period. We generally recommend that punishments last 1–3 minutes times the age of the child, depending on the severity of the infraction (i.e., about 10 to 30 minutes for a child who is age 10). Ideally, punishment is combined with very brief instruction given to the child on the behavior they are expected to perform. Engage parents in a discussion of these principles.

- "What principles should you keep in mind to help punishment work effectively?"
- "How can you be consistent in using punishment?"
- "Why is it important to deliver punishment immediately after a target behavior occurs?"

- "What does it mean to be *specific* in delivering punishment?"
- "What does it mean to be *salient* in delivering punishment?"
- "How long should a punishment last for your child?"
- "What are the disadvantages of long punishments?"
- "How can you be sure you teach appropriate behavior along with giving a punishment?"

3.c. *Discuss strategies parents can use to maintain emotional control when punishing their child.* Engage parents in a discussion of why it is important to maintain emotional control when punishing. Parents typically have excellent strategies for maintaining control, but often have difficulty implementing these in the heat of the moment.

- "Why is it important to maintain emotional control when punishing your child?"
- "What strategies do you use to keep emotional control?"
- "How consistently do you use these strategies?"
- "What could you do to remind yourself to use these strategies more consistently?"
- "How could another caregiver help you be more consistent in maintaining emotional control?"

3.d. *Help parents understand how they should behave during and after punishment.* Parents often make the mistake of getting highly involved with their child during punishment. The problem with this is that parents are giving positive reinforcement (i.e., parental attention) to children when they are being punished, which sends a mixed message. Emphasize the importance of remaining disengaged with their child during and shortly after punishment. During punishment parents should briefly state the reason for the punishment. No other comment is needed. After punishment is over, the parent should get back into the mode of trying to catch the child being good.

- "What is the best approach for parents to use when their child is being punished?"
- "What should you say to your child while your child is being punished?"
- "What should you do after punishment is over?"
- "When is a good time to have a discussion with your child about why they were punished?"

Pro Tip

Some parents prefer to have a lengthy discussion about why the child was punished after the punishment is over. If parents want to have this discussion, we recommend that it takes place well after the punishment is over, so the child does not get parental attention close in time to the punishment period.

Goal 4—Assign homework and identify practice supports for consistent implementation. (5 minutes)

- *Request that parents engage children in a discussion about how punishment will be used.* Encourage parents to work with their child to delineate important family rules and identify two behaviors that will be punished when these occur. In addition, encourage parents to dis-

Session 8: Using Punishment Successfully 111

cuss with their child what the punishment will be when these targeted behaviors occur. Ask parents to complete the Homework—*Using Punishment Strategically* worksheet.

- *Encourage parents to practice using punishment for the identified target behaviors.* Encourage parents to remember principles of effective punishment (consistency, immediacy, specificity, saliency, 4:1 ratio; CISS-4) and to remain calm when implementing punishment.
- *Encourage parents to keep working on the goal-setting strategy.* Ask parents to bring completed goal-setting worksheets to the next session.
- *Encourage parents to keep implementing Child's Game.*
- *Encourage parents to call you if any questions or concerns arise in the coming week.*

Session 8 Child Group Agenda

1. Review the group rules and token reinforcement system.
2. Maintain group cohesion.
3. Discuss experience and progress with homework goal-setting strategies.
4. Discuss appropriate consequences for unproductive and disruptive behavior.
5. Conclude session.

Materials Needed

- For token reinforcement system—stopwatch/timer (for keeping track of 15-minute intervals) and flip chart
- Name tags
- Deck of playing cards
- Crayons/markers
- Cards for Concentration Game
- Reinforcers that can be used as part of a token reinforcement system
- Snacks for snack break during session

Goal 1—Review the group rules and token reinforcement system.

Escort children into the child therapy room after a brief, joint orientation with their parents. The first goal is to make sure children are oriented to the group rules that were developed during the initial session and the token reinforcement system.

- Remind children of the group name they agreed on during the initial session.
- Ask children to identify rules that were identified during the initial session.
- Review how the token economy operates and ask children if they have any questions.

- Review the agenda for the current session and activities.
- Start the first 15-minute interval for the token reinforcement system.

Goal 2—Maintain group cohesion.

Work on maintaining group cohesion. Building group cohesion was an important part of the initial sessions. In subsequent group sessions, it is important for group leaders to dedicate some time to maintaining good relationships among the group members.

- Ask each child what they liked best about the most recent group session. Each child should be encouraged to talk about at least one thing they enjoyed.
- Ask children to share their favorite holiday and a reason why this holiday is their favorite. Praise children for participating. Encourage children to share additional thoughts about their favorite holidays.

Goal 3—Discuss experience and progress with homework goal-setting strategies.

The goal of this portion of the child group session is to provide children with an opportunity to share their experiences with the homework goal-setting strategy. Because the goal-setting strategy can be challenging at first for many families, providing children with an opportunity to discuss their experience and ask questions can support improvements with implementation.

- Ask children to share their experience with practicing the goal-setting strategies with their parents.
- Engage children in talking about whether they are doing homework differently and, if so, how.
- Engage children in a role-play activity to practice the homework goal-setting strategy (using the same approach as Session 7).
- Prepare children for the upcoming break, by explaining that all rules still apply, and describing how children will take turns going to the bathroom.

Snack Break

Goal 4—Discuss appropriate consequences for unproductive and disruptive behavior.

Similar to Session 6 (discussion of homework experiences), the discussion about consequences is supported by using a Concentration Game designed to help children feel comfortable sharing their thoughts and feelings. The rules and process for the game are the same as Session 6, but the focus is now on consequences.

- Prior to the session, the group leader should create a set of Concentration Game cards. One side of each card should have a question or statement written on it about positive reinforcement and punishment (e.g., What do your parents do when you pay attention and work hard while you are completing your homework; What do your parents do when you do not work hard during homework time?). The cards should be created in pairs, with each pair including the same question/statement. Other pairs of cards with pictures (such as animals, smiling faces, common objects) should be created as well. Cards can be the size of one-half of a 3 × 5 index card.
- Have the children sit in a circle while the group leader places the cards face down in a random order to form a square grid.
- One by one, each child is instructed to choose two cards that are identical to each other (i.e., have the same question or same picture). The child gets a point if they either adequately answer a question or pick a pair of pictures. All children are encouraged to answer the question.

Goal 5—Conclude session.

- Engage children in a card game or art activity, according to their choice, if there is time remaining.
- Announce point totals and allow children to choose prizes. Emphasize positive behaviors displayed by each child. Do not focus on disruptive behaviors. Rather, encourage the children to keep up the effort to follow rules throughout the week and at the next session.

CHAPTER 13

FSS Session 9
Planning for Future Success

Session 9 Agenda

1. Review homework assigned at last session with a focus on consistent implementation. (25 minutes)
2. Support parents in applying FSS strategies to challenging situations. (25 minutes)
3. Guide parents in developing their individual "Formula for Success." (30 minutes)
4. Celebrate families' completion of FSS. (10 minutes)

Materials Needed

- Handout—*How to Address Challenging Situations*
- Handout—*Challenging Situations Worksheet* (for completion during session)
- Handout—*Maintaining Success and Anticipating Future Problems*
- Handout—*Formula for Success*
- Handout—*Finding a Provider for Behavior Management with ADHD*
- Handout—*Certificate of Completion* (one for each family)
- Handout—*Template for Report of Progress*
- Handouts (or posters)—*FSS Theory of Change* and *Attention Grid* (both distributed in Session 1)
- Dry-erase markers (to post agenda on whiteboard with time limits for each section if in-person session)

Session Process Reminders

1. Focus on using open-ended questions.
2. Practice reflective listening throughout session to highlight and build on key points.
3. Validate emotions parents are experiencing related to their parenting.
4. Affirm parents for any effort or movement in the direction of change and implementation of recommended strategies.
5. Support all parents in participating, but avoid putting anyone on the spot.
6. Facilitate the group interacting with each other, rather than just the clinician(s).
7. Keep the group focused on key points and refocus the discussion if it becomes tangential.

Goal 1—Review homework assigned at the last session with a focus on consistent implementation. (25 minutes)

The homework assigned at the end of Session 8 asked parents to engage their children in a discussion about using punishment, including establishing key "house rules" to help the child understand behaviors that will be punished. Additionally, parents were encouraged to identify the punishments that will be used and to practice using punishment when target behaviors occurred. Homework also included continuing to work on refining the homework goal-setting strategy. Finally, there should be a brief check in with the parents about continuing to use Child's Game.

Collect completed homework assignments and make copies. Continue to emphasize the importance of completing homework assignments. Encourage parents to share how they receive support from other caregivers in implementing homework assignments.

1.a. *Encourage parents to discuss their experiences using punishment.* The main focus of homework review should be on supporting parents in sharing their experiences applying punishment strategies in response to target behaviors. It is important for the discussion to focus on identifying appropriate target behaviors for punishment, being consistent in applying punishment, and maintaining emotional control when applying punishment strategies.

- "What was your experience discussing the use of punishment with your child?"
- "What 'house rules' did you establish?"
- "What behaviors did you identify as targets for punishment?"
- "What types of punishment strategies are you using?"
- "What strategies are you using to remain calm when using punishment?"
- "What challenges have you encountered using punishment?"

1.b. *Ask parents to share their experiences with continuing to use homework goal setting.* This should be a relatively brief check-in with parents to affirm their ongoing efforts with this strategy and answer any questions about challenges to successful implementation.

- "How is homework goal setting going?"
- "What changes are you seeing in homework completion?"
- "How have you responded to any challenges experienced with homework goal setting?"

1.c. *Discuss parents' experiences in implementing Child's Game.* Focus on and affirm efforts parents have made to continue using this strategy.

- "What activities are you doing for Child's Game?"
- "What are some of the challenges with continuing to use Child's Game each day?"

Goal 2—Support parents in applying FSS strategies to challenging situations. (25 minutes)

This section provides an opportunity to support parents in applying FSS principles and strategies to situations that have not been discussed previously. At this point in the program, parents have the foundation needed to address unresolved problems and unforeseen challenges that lie ahead. This section of the session enables parents to review the A-B-C model for analyzing problems and planning an alternative approach to parenting their child. In addition, this section provides parents an opportunity to address two especially challenging situations: (1) using punishment when children are highly dysregulated emotionally and behaviorally, and (2) managing behavior in public settings.

2.a. *Help parents develop an overall framework for addressing challenging behaviors and situations.* The overall purpose of this part of the session is to encourage integration and generalization of strategies. Distribute the handouts *Challenging Situations* and *Challenging Situations Worksheet* to facilitate the discussion and support parents in developing an approach to managing challenging situations in the future. Through this discussion, parents should develop a framework to (1) identify the problem (the "not-OK behavior"), (2) identify the more desired replacement behavior (the "OK behavior"), (3) think about the ABC's of the desired and problematic behaviors, (4) modify the antecedents to increase the probability of the desired behavior, (5) identify ways to use positive reinforcement, (6) determine if punishment or ignoring strategies are needed, and (7) consider factors that can support consistent use of techniques. The clinician can ask if a parent is continuing to struggle with a challenging situation and use this as an example of how to apply A-B-C strategies to solve problems in the future.

- "What could you do when faced with a behavior or situation you have not previously managed?"
- "What are key behavioral change strategies that parents should consider when developing a plan to address challenging situations or behavior?"
- "How can you tell when your plan is effective?"
- "Who is willing to describe a situation you are continuing to struggle with? Let's work together to come up with a plan to address this situation. How should we approach this?"

Pro Tip

This exercise is designed to promote group collaborative problem solving. Clinicians should try to resist the tendency for this to be an individualized activity between the clinician and the parent who presents the challenging situation.

2.b. *Discuss strategies for using punishment with children when they are dysregulated.* Delivering punishment when a child is dysregulated can trigger a strong emotional reaction (e.g., severe and extended temper tantrum). When children are in this state, we generally recommend that parents use ignoring instead of punishment to address the situation. However, at times ignoring is not an appropriate response, such as when the child has been aggressive with a sibling. When punishment is needed, the parent can issue a verbal correction and ensure that no family member gives attention to the child, while maintaining control of their own emotions. The period of punishment (time out from family attention) can be relatively brief, but no one in the family should reengage until the child begins to calm down. Some children have extreme difficulty calming down during punishment, resulting in tantrums that can last for well over an hour and be highly disruptive to family routines. In these cases, parents may need to provide coaching to the child, giving prompts for self-control and praising any efforts the child makes to calm down. If coaching is needed, it is important for parents to provide the minimal amount of attention needed to assist the child in gaining control.

- "When your child is having a bad day, what do you do when your child violates family rules?"
- "In these situations, when is it appropriate to use ignoring versus punishment?"
- "If punishment is needed, how can you implement this?"
- "What do you do if your child has a severe temper tantrum while being punished?"
- "What should you do if your child does not calm down for a long period of time after being punished?"

Pro Tip

Parents who struggle in implementing punishment with dysregulated children often need a referral for individualized family behavior therapy.

2.c. *Assist parents in planning for how to manage behavior in public places.* The key to promoting children's success in public places is to focus on antecedent conditions. Parents should have realistic expectations for the amount of time a child can maintain self-control in a public place. It is important for parents to remind children of a few essential rules of behavior before entering the public place. Parents should be prepared to catch children following these rules on a frequent basis and may want to give tokens or points to children when they follow rules in these situations. When children misbehave in public places, the use of ignoring and targeted verbal corrections are generally recommended. If a more potent punishment is needed, parents can consider using a brief time out, which could involve leaving the public place and placing the child in an obscure place or in the car for a very brief period of time while being carefully supervised.

- "What is a reasonable amount of time for your child to spend in public places?"
- "How can you be prepared to set your child up for success in a public place?"
- "How could you use your token system in a public place?"
- "How do you want to respond to child misbehavior when in public?"
- "If a time out is needed, how can you implement this in a public place?"

Goal 3—Guide parents in developing their individual "Formula for Success." (30 minutes)

To conclude the program, parents are provided an opportunity to develop an individualized plan to strengthen the parent–child relationship, establish and sustain meaningful family–school partnerships, and address challenging situations that arise at home and school. The purpose is to guide parents in identifying strategies they have found most helpful and feasible to use. This culminates with parents writing their "Formula for Success," which essentially serves as the family's "playbook" to promote their child's success at home and school. Parents are encouraged to develop their Formula for Success with their child.

3.a. *Provide parents an opportunity to identify the most helpful FSS strategies.* As an initial step in developing the Formula for Success, ask parents to briefly identify the strategies that they have found most useful over the course of FSS. Parents should also be encouraged to share with other group members how they may have adapted strategies to work well in their family. Clinicians should use the handout *Maintaining Success and Anticipating Future Problems* to guide a brief review of the main components of FSS.

- "What strategies were the most important to you and helped you the most?"
- "How did you adapt strategies to make them work better in your household?"

3.b. *Guide parents in developing their individual Formula for Success.* Creating a Formula for Success helps parents reflect on FSS strategies that have been most helpful for them. Each family's Formula for Success may emphasize different strategies. Use the handout *Formula for Success* to help guide the discussion. Give parents a few minutes to reflect on the worksheet privately, and then encourage them to share their Formula for Success with the rest of the group. The clinician may need to encourage parents to identify strategies for both home and school. The clinician should discuss with parents how they will remember to review and apply their Formula for Success when things are not going well. In addition, the clinician should emphasize the importance of staying connected with other parents to weather the difficult times and maintain consistent use of FSS strategies.

- "What are your go-to strategies to promote your child's success at home and school?"
- "What strategies do you think will be the most helpful when you face new situations in the future?"
- "How can you remember your Formula for Success when you need it?"
- "How can you involve your child in further developing your Formula for Success?"
- "How can you stay connected with other families in the future to sustain the gains you have made during the program?"

Pro Tip

To sustain the gains of the FSS program, it is important for parents to establish and maintain partnerships with other parents who are coping with similar challenges. As such, we strongly recommend referring families to local parent support groups.

Goal 4—Celebrate families' completion of FSS. (10 minutes)

The clinician should use this as an opportunity to recognize and affirm parents for their engagement and effort during the FSS program. The clinician should highlight the efforts parents have made to connect with and support one another during this process. It is important to note that ADHD is a chronic condition and that families typically need psychosocial intervention at various points during the child's development. Encourage parents to get involved in care when they anticipate their child and family may be facing a challenging period. It is possible one or more families may need individualized psychosocial intervention after the program ends. In these cases, the clinician can help the family access additional care in their practice or make referrals for services in the community. Some clinicians and families may find the guidance summarized in the handout *Finding a Provider for Behavior Management with ADHD* helpful in identifying clinicians appropriately trained and experienced in providing care for individuals with ADHD. The session concludes with the clinician distributing a *Certificate of Completion* to each of the families. If the clinician is planning to provide a summary of program outcomes to families, we suggest using the handout *Template for Report of Progress*, as described in Chapter 16 and included in Appendix A.

Session 9 Child Group Agenda

1. Review the group rules and token reinforcement system.
2. Maintain group cohesion.
3. Discuss the parts of the program children found helpful.
4. Celebrate completion of FSS.
5. Conclude session.

Materials Needed

- For token reinforcement system—stopwatch/timer (for keeping track of 15-minute intervals) and flip chart
- Name tags
- Deck of playing cards
- Crayons/markers
- Reinforcers that can be used as part of a token reinforcement system
- Snacks for snack break during session

Goal 1—Review the group rules and token reinforcement system.

Escort children into the child therapy room after a brief, joint orientation with their parents. The first goal is to make sure the children are oriented to the group rules that were developed during the initial session and the token reinforcement system.

- Remind children of the group name they agreed on during the initial session.
- Ask children to identify rules that were identified during the initial session.
- Review how the token economy operates and ask children if they have any questions.
- Review the agenda for the current session and activities.
- Start the first 15-minute interval for the token reinforcement system.

Goal 2—Maintain group cohesion.

Work on maintaining group cohesion. Building group cohesion was an important part of the initial sessions. In subsequent group sessions, it is important for group leaders to dedicate some time to maintaining good relationships among the group members.

- Ask each child what they liked best about the most recent group session. Each child should be encouraged to talk about at least one thing they enjoyed.

Goal 3—Discuss the parts of the program children found helpful.

The goal of this portion of the child group session is to support children in identifying the components of FSS they have found helpful. This will parallel the discussion that is occurring in the parent group, as the parents are developing their individual "Formula for Success."

- Ask children to identify things their parents are doing that are different than before FSS.
- Ask children to share one strategy that they think is particularly helpful.
- Support children in identifying what about homework and family relationships they would like to see improved in the future.
- Ask children to share how they can use strategies their family has learned to make future improvements.
- Prepare children for the upcoming break, by explaining that all rules still apply, and describing how children will take turns going to the bathroom.

Snack Break

Goal 4—Celebrate completion of FSS.

Group leaders should use this as an opportunity to recognize children for their participation and effort throughout the program. Group leaders should emphasize active participation in group activities, completing role plays, and following the group rules developed at the start of the program. It is also important to help children reflect on how their effort in the program resulted in improvements at home and school.

Goal 5—Conclude session.

- Engage children in a card game or art activity, according to their choice, if there is time remaining.
- Announce point totals and allow children to choose prizes. Emphasize positive behaviors displayed by each child. Do not focus on disruptive behaviors. Rather, encourage the children to keep up the effort to follow rules throughout the week and into the future.

SECTION III

ADAPTATIONS AND EVALUATION

CHAPTER 14

Adaptations across Settings, Populations, and Time of Year

FSS was designed for delivery predominantly as a group intervention in schools and outpatient behavioral health clinic settings with families of children in grades 1–5. Chapters 3 and 4 provide detailed information about how to set up groups and conduct sessions. This includes strategies for recruiting families, implementing FSS in schools and mental health clinic settings, including children in sessions, and delivering each session successfully in an organized and efficient manner.

In addition to implementation in schools and mental health clinics, FSS can be implemented in a range of other settings (e.g., primary care practices, private practice), in person and using telehealth, and individually with families (rather than in groups). Additionally, FSS strategies can readily be adapted for younger children and with greater effort adapted for older students, with developmentally appropriate modifications. Adaptations also might be helpful when working with parents with diverse family constellations. In addition, as noted throughout this book, FSS includes a strong focus on fostering collaborative family–school partnerships. The strategies described in previous chapters are useful when FSS is offered while school is in session; adaptations are necessary when FSS is offered during the summer months. This chapter includes suggestions for delivering FSS in different situations and contexts, including:

- How can I deliver FSS in primary care?
- How can I offer FSS in private practice?
- Can telehealth be used to deliver FSS?
- Can I offer FSS in individual family sessions?
- How do I modify FSS for use with families of young children?
- How do I modify FSS for use with families of older students?
- What modifications are necessary when offering FSS in the summer?
- What considerations should I keep in mind when working with varying family constellations?

HOW CAN I DELIVER FSS IN PRIMARY CARE?

Integration of behavioral health into primary care practices is one effective method for increasing accessibility and utilization of services, reducing stigma related to mental health services, and reducing health disparities (Asarnow et al., 2015; Shahidullah et al., 2023). In these models of care, patients and families receive behavioral health care in the same setting as their primary health care. Integrated behavioral health models include fully integrated (i.e., behavioral health clinician operates as a core member of the care team) and co-located approaches (i.e., behavioral health clinician works within the same clinic but operates somewhat separately from the primary care team; Asarnow et al., 2017). When delivered in integrated primary care clinics, BPT programs result in improved child and family outcomes and more equitable access to care (Smith et al., 2020).

Similar to other BPT programs implemented in primary care, FSS is likely to be feasible for integrated behavioral health clinicians to deliver in primary care practices. In this case, referrals are likely to originate from primary care clinicians (i.e., physicians, nurse practitioners) or other members of the care team (e.g., nurses, psychologists, psychiatrists, licensed clinical social workers). Primary care clinicians might make referrals after hearing from families if schools have concerns about the child's academic performance. Additionally, parents might self-refer if they are aware that FSS is available in their child's primary care practice.

One of the benefits of implementing FSS in primary care is the opportunity to include collaboration with the child's primary care clinician throughout the program. Given that treatment guidelines typically suggest a combination of medication and behavioral intervention for treatment of school-age children with ADHD (Wolraich et al., 2019) and that primary care clinicians frequently manage ADHD medications, collaboration between behavioral health clinicians integrated into primary care practices and primary care clinicians is highly beneficial for youth with ADHD (e.g., Kolko et al., 2014; Power et al., 2014). For example, behavioral health clinicians might be able to assist with monitoring response to medication treatment and support family adherence to medication treatment plans (Shahidullah et al., 2018). Additionally, clinicians leading the FSS program in primary care can support collaborations between the family, the school, and the health system. This type of multisystemic collaboration can result in improved outcomes for children and families coping with ADHD (Power, Blum, et al., 2013).

Other than issues related to participant recruitment and collaboration between FSS clinicians and primary care clinicians, implementation of FSS in primary care practices is likely to be very similar to implementation in behavioral health clinic settings. Strategies for setting up the program and conducting sessions described in Chapters 3 and 4 are highly applicable to implementation in primary care.

HOW CAN I OFFER FSS IN PRIVATE PRACTICE?

Practitioners who work in private practices serving children and families are likely to work with many children with ADHD and related difficulties. Given the high demand for behavioral health services, private practitioners are likely to receive many requests for appointments, and delivery of FSS to groups of families might be an efficient way to support multiple families at once. That said, if the practice is small or has limited administrative infrastructure, recruitment and scheduling of groups could be challenging. As a result, private practitioners might find delivery of FSS to families individually to be more feasible (see the section on delivery in individualized sessions below for suggestions for offering FSS to individual families).

Practitioners in private practice who offer FSS in groups might have to develop recruitment pathways to identify families interested in participating in the program. The practitioner might consider sending a communication to all potentially eligible families on their caseload about the group offering, advertising with local parenting groups (e.g., through social media platforms), and accepting referrals from other mental health practitioners or health care providers in the community or from local schools.

It might be challenging for practitioners in private practice to collaborate with schools. We encourage practitioners to attempt to develop relationships with local schools whenever possible. Identifying an individual in each school who might serve as a "behavioral health champion" (e.g., guidance counselor, school psychologist, school social worker), is a helpful way to initiate a partnership. Then, as the practitioner engages in school collaboration for each family in the group, the school-based champion might be able to help facilitate connections with the children's teachers. This could also lead to future referrals for the program. Before initiating communication with local schools related to any individual child, practitioners are encouraged to follow the guidelines in Chapter 4 related to obtaining consent to communicate with schools/teachers.

CAN TELEHEALTH BE USED TO DELIVER FSS?

It is highly feasible to offer group parent-focused programs for families coping with ADHD via telehealth (Fogler et al., 2020). In fact, there are clear advantages to offering FSS using telehealth, perhaps most notably that it substantially decreases the amount of time it takes families to participate in the intervention because they do not need to travel to sessions. Related, families usually do not need to be concerned about arranging for child care in order to attend sessions. As such, telehealth service delivery may reduce the financial costs to families. In making adaptations to ensure high-quality intervention delivery via telehealth, we strongly recommend that clinicians attend carefully to process fidelity dimensions (see Chapter 15 and Appendix B; see also Fogler et al., 2020).

There are several noteworthy challenges to delivering FSS using telehealth. First, it may not be feasible for families to participate for 90 minutes per session when they attend virtually. We typically offer our group telehealth sessions in 75 minutes, which can make it difficult to address all of the session content using the dialogic approach recommended for this intervention. We recommend that practitioners resist the tendency to make sessions more didactic in order to address all elements of the session. Instead, we suggest they determine beforehand which sections will be shortened and how to limit the length of time for discussion. Second, some families experience technological difficulties when participating in sessions virtually. Families marginalized by lower-income status may be especially vulnerable to interruptions due to technological challenges. It is important to spend time collaborating with families before the first session and throughout the program, resolving these issues to minimize disruptions that interfere with family engagement. Third, it can be challenging to facilitate connections among family members in the group when using telehealth. Our practitioners who use telehealth to deliver parent groups usually need to make a concerted effort to prompt parents to share comments with one another and reduce the number of comments made directly to practitioners.

Our team has noted that in some telehealth groups there is a tendency for parents to turn off cameras during sessions. This pattern often gets established early in the program; one or two parents turn off their cameras during the first session and by the middle of the program several parents have their cameras turned off for most of the session. This pattern can be highly detrimental to promoting family engagement and motivation. We strongly recommend that practitioners indicate clearly at the outset the importance of participating with cameras on, acknowledging that it may be necessary for parents to turn off their cameras briefly during a session.

Including children can be challenging during virtual sessions. We sometimes involve children at the outset of meetings to discuss progress and implementation of strategies during the past week. We involve children during the latter parts of Session 2 (Child's Game), Session 5 (token reinforcement), and Session 7 (goal setting and time management) so the parent(s) and child can practice the strategies or have a discussion during the session. If there are two or more practitioners (including trainees) conducting the session, it is often helpful to separate parents into subgroups to practice strategies and for a clinician to join each subgroup, as long as the videoconferencing platform being used allows for this feature.

Adaptations are usually needed to model FSS strategies during virtual sessions. One approach is to show brief videos to parents that provide illustrations of how to implement strategies, such as Child's Game. Videos can be prepared by practitioners or downloaded from websites that provide useful training to parents. For example, YouTube includes videos that might be useful to demonstrate some FSS strategies. It is recommended that practitioners carefully review any online content prior to sharing with the group to ensure that the examples are of high quality and appropriate. Alternatively, if there are two practitioners, parents can observe them implementing the strategy in a role play.

CAN I OFFER FSS IN INDIVIDUALIZED FAMILY SESSIONS?

The FSS program can be adapted quite readily for implementation in individualized family therapy sessions rather than in groups. Clear advantages are the ability to tailor sessions to address the unique needs of each family and numerous opportunities to involve children in sessions to engage in role plays and guided practice implementing FSS strategies with feedback from the practitioner. This might be particularly useful for families in which the child is experiencing a high level of impairment and individualized attention is warranted. For example, the practitioner might first demonstrate how to engage in Child's Game with the child, and then the parent(s) and child could practice the strategy together. The practitioner can offer live feedback on implementation.

Individualized family sessions might also be useful for families in which the parents need focused support to address challenges with co-parenting. Individualized discussions about the parenting partnership and approaches to strategy implementation might be more comfortable than group discussions for parents experiencing co-parenting challenges.

In addition, it may be feasible to schedule individualized family sessions at a time that enables school professionals to participate virtually, affording opportunities for conjoint family–school consultation (Sheridan & Kratochwill, 2007). As noted above, individualized family sessions might also be more feasible for practitioners working in private practice, who may have limited infrastructure to support recruitment and scheduling for groups.

When conducting individualized sessions, we typically recommend shortening the sessions to 45–50 minutes. Because individualized sessions do not include group discussion of content, sessions will naturally be shorter. That said, it is important for practitioners offering individualized sessions to plan ahead and determine the schedule/agenda for each session to ensure that key points are addressed. Even though the session will not include group discussion, practitioners should avoid the tendency to deliver the content in a didactic manner. If more than one caregiver is present, those caregivers can be encouraged to discuss the content together.

A noteworthy limitation of not including other families is that parents do not have opportunities to connect with other parents and obtain support from them, which facilitates the process of self-empowerment. In addition, parents do not have the opportunity to learn from other parents and build confidence by sharing their ideas with other parents and being affirmed by them. When determining whether to provide individualized or group-based care, clinicians might engage in a shared decision-making process with families, highlighting benefits and drawbacks of each approach and encouraging parents to share their perspectives about the options.

HOW DO I MODIFY FSS FOR USE WITH FAMILIES OF YOUNG CHILDREN?

Although FSS was designed primarily for children in grades 1–5, the big ideas and main principles of FSS (i.e., focus on strengthening relationships and modifying environmental contingencies to encourage appropriate behavior) are applicable to kindergarten- and preschool-age children as well. That said, it is important for clinicians to work with families to ensure that FSS strategies are modified in developmentally appropriate ways for young children. For example, preschoolers might require more frequent reinforcement schedules than children in elementary school do. Clinicians working with families of younger children might focus on developing token economies that result in multiple opportunities per day for children to earn rewards, especially in the beginning.

In addition, because children below first grade usually are not assigned homework by teachers, adaptations of sessions focused on homework (Sessions 6 and 7) are typically necessary. We recommend that clinicians work with parents to identify educational activities they engage in with their children at home, such as reading books together, playing a simple card or board game, baking cookies, and identifying signs on the road. These activities are homework for young children and can be substituted for teacher-assigned homework in adapting some of the FSS sessions. Maintaining this focus on educational activities at home with younger children encourages family involvement in education and sets the stage for formal learning opportunities as children enter elementary school.

HOW DO I MODIFY FSS FOR USE WITH FAMILIES OF OLDER STUDENTS?

Over the years, we have received feedback from many families that FSS does not address some of needs of students in middle school and above. Although the big ideas and main principles of FSS are applicable to older students, most of the examples provided in this guidebook are more appropriate for younger children. For example, adolescents may be more motivated by spending time outside the home with peers and engaging with friends using social media. In addition, adolescents typically want more input into designing rewards systems than younger children do. It is usually important to work on communication and negotiation strategies with parents and adolescents, so they can collaborate to solve problems and develop behavior-change strategies, such as behavioral contracts.

Students in grade 6 and above, and often those as young as in grade 3, benefit from direct skills training to improve organization, time management, and planning skills, which are required for successful performance of independent activities, such as homework and performing multistep chores (Evans et al., 2016; Sibley et al., 2016). We strongly recommend that family–school interventions for students in middle school and above include a focus on youth skills training, in addition to behavioral parent training and school collaboration. In addition, motivational interviewing with students and parents can be beneficial to promote motivation and engagement in intervention (Sibley et al., 2016).

WHAT MODIFICATIONS ARE NECESSARY WHEN OFFERING FSS IN THE SUMMER?

Program modifications are needed in offering FSS at the end of the school year and during the summer when students may not be attending school and getting homework assignments. An adaptation we have made at the end of the academic year is to discuss how to prepare for the following school year, including establishing partnerships with teachers, developing a daily report card, establishing a useful homework routine, and implementing time management and goal-setting strategies during homework. Even if teachers have reduced homework assignments at the end of the school year, parents can identify homework activities for their children, such as engaging in independent reading or completing a worksheet from one of their texts, and work on implementing homework strategies with these tasks.

Our team usually does not offer FSS during the early and middle parts of the summer, although the program may have utility in midsummer if children are in summer school or involved in a summer camp that includes educational programming. Starting FSS at the end of the summer is often feasible and helpful for families. We often start FSS 2 weeks before the start of school, so the fourth session, which is focused on school collaboration, occurs when children have been in school for about a week, and the sixth and seventh sessions, focused on student homework performance, occur when students have been in school for 3 or 4 weeks. There are real advantages to starting FSS early in the school year, including establishing a collaborative partnership with teachers and establishing homework and family routines that promote student organization and productivity before unproductive patterns and conflictual relationships are established.

WHAT CONSIDERATIONS SHOULD I KEEP IN MIND WHEN WORKING WITH VARYING FAMILY CONSTELLATIONS?

Over the years, we have conducted FSS groups with families with a range of family constellations, including two-working-parent households, families with a parent who does not work outside the home, single-parent households, multigenerational families, extended families, and blended families. Parenting children with ADHD is challenging; parents need the support of other caregivers, family, and friends to obtain the resources and strength to cope successfully and be effective in using positive parenting approaches. It is critical that clinicians encourage all parents, regardless of family composition, to identify ways to obtain the support they need from other adults in the child's life. Some families might determine that it makes sense to ask additional caregivers to join FSS sessions; we encourage this so parents and other caregivers can work together to learn strategies and develop plans to implement them consistently.

CONCLUSIONS

FSS was developed for implementation in schools and outpatient behavioral health clinic settings. The intervention can be adapted for use in primary care, private practice, and by telehealth. FSS is designed for delivery with groups of families, but it also can be adapted as an individualized family intervention. Because of the focus on child homework, family involvement in education, and collaborative family–school relationships, the program is typically provided during the school year, but adjustments can be made for delivery during the summer months. In addition, FSS can be readily adapted for use with children in preschool and kindergarten, as described above. More substantial modifications are necessary for youth in grades 6 and above. Finally, given the strong focus in FSS on parent coping and organization and on strengthening caregiver–child relationships, it is critically important to promote strong networks of caregiving support among families with diverse constellations.

CHAPTER 15

Assessing Intervention Fidelity, Engagement, and Outcomes

with Jenelle Nissley-Tsiopinis

An essential part of the FSS program is evaluating the outcomes of the intervention and exploring factors that may be contributing to favorable or unfavorable outcomes. In this chapter we describe a plan for program evaluation guided by the FSS theory of change illustrated in Chapter 2. The plan has a major focus on assessing child outcomes in the home and school settings related to homework performance, academic performance, other areas of functioning (impairment), symptoms of ADHD, and internalizing and externalizing behaviors. In addition, the evaluation plan includes an examination of potential mechanisms of action or proximal variables that may serve to mediate the effect of FSS on child outcomes (e.g., parenting practices). Further, the evaluation plan includes strategies for assessing how FSS is implemented by providers (fidelity) and how it is received by participants (engagement), which is useful in determining the extent to which families have actually obtained FSS as designed.

This chapter describes recommended procedures for assessing fidelity and engagement, proximal outcomes, and child outcomes at home and school. Recommended measures, sources of data, and timelines for data collection are described in Table 15.1. The chapter includes sections describing:

- Measures of intervention fidelity and engagement
- Measures of family and family–school relationship outcomes
- Measures of child outcomes
- Measure of program satisfaction

Jenelle Nissley-Tsiopinis, PhD, is a research and clinical psychologist at the Center for the Management of ADHD at Children's Hospital of Philadelphia.

TABLE 15.1. List of Potential Measures and Recommended Timeline for Data Collection

Measure/evaluation	Source of data	Preintervention	During intervention	Postintervention
Measures of fidelity and engagement				
FSS practitioner content fidelity	FSS practitioner/observer		X	
FSS practitioner process fidelity	FSS practitioner/observer		X	
FSS program session attendance	FSS practitioner		X	
Ratings of parent completion of between-session homework	FSS practitioner		X	
Coding of parent completion of between-session homework	FSS practitioner		X	
Measures of proximal outcomes				
Parent–Child Relationship Questionnaire	Parent	X		X
Parent–Teacher Involvement Questionnaire	Parent, teacher	X		X
Parent as Educator Scale	Parent	X		X
Measures of distal, child outcomes				
Behavioral Health Checklist	Parent	X		X
Homework Performance Questionnaire—Parent	Parent	X		X
Homework Problem Checklist	Parent	X		X
Impairment Rating Scale—Parent	Parent	X		X
Homework Performance Questionnaire—Teacher	Teacher	X		X
Impairment Rating Scale—Teacher	Teacher	X		X
Academic Proficiency Scale	Teacher	X		X
Measure of FSS program satisfaction				
Program Evaluation Scale	Parent			X

In the final chapter (Chapter 16), we provide case examples that illustrate how to utilize the measures in a clinical context to evaluate individual family outcomes (e.g., to identify families who require additional support after FSS and who may benefit from individualized follow-up treatment).

MEASURES OF INTERVENTION FIDELITY AND ENGAGEMENT

Many factors contribute to the effectiveness of an intervention; two key factors are implementation fidelity and participant engagement. Fidelity can be broken down into the components, steps, or content of intervention (content fidelity) and the competence or process by which the intervention is delivered (process fidelity). Engagement can be differentiated into dosage of intervention received (attendance) and extent of practice with intervention skills (adherence to between-session homework assignments; Power et al., 2005). This section describes methods we recommend for assessing content and process fidelity as well as family engagement in FSS.

Content Fidelity

It is perhaps self-evident that achieving successful outcomes depends to some extent on whether the components (content) of an intervention are actually delivered by providers. Examining content fidelity is relatively straightforward and consists of recording whether each element has been implemented. The main challenge with assessing content fidelity is identifying the key components of each session and including one or more items aligned with each component. Content fidelity can be assessed by self-reports, although these may provide overestimates of implementation. A more accurate way of examining content fidelity is for external observers to conduct the assessment. Observations can be conducted directly in real time or through ratings of audio/video recordings of sessions. The content fidelity forms we use for FSS request providers or observers to indicate whether each element of an FSS session was implemented or was not implemented. When content fidelity is assessed using both self-reports and external ratings, it can provide a useful opportunity for collaboration and performance feedback for the provider. We recommend that external reviews occur with the informed consent of the intervention provider.

Process Fidelity

Although implementing the components of FSS is critically important, it is just as important to deliver the intervention competently and with high quality. In our group parent training work related to the Bootcamp for ADHD program, we have identified five critical process fidelity dimensions (Fogler et al., 2020; Nissley-Tsiopinis et al., 2023). The process dimensions highlight the importance of delivering the intervention in a manner that is responsive to the unique, culturally influenced circumstances of each participating family, facilitates a process of self-empowerment, and promotes adaptation of the intervention to unique family circumstances. We have found these dimensions to be highly applicable in implementing the FSS program. The following is a description of each dimension and procedures for evaluating process fidelity when FSS is delivered in a group context with several parents. See Table 15.2 for examples of questions and comments clinicians can make that are aligned with each process dimension.

TABLE 15.2. Process Fidelity Dimensions: Description and Examples

Process fidelity dimension	Description of dimension	Examples of practitioner comments that align with the dimension
Encouraging parent active engagement	Clinician uses open-ended questions, affirmations, reflections, and summaries to encourage parent engagement; clinician adapts material to individual parent situations.	"What behaviors would you like your child to change?" "What happens before that behavior occurs that might set your child up for failure or misbehavior?"
Eliciting and strengthening change talk	Clinician elicits and affirms parents' desire, ability, reasons and need for change.	"It sounds like you would like to have a more collaborative relationship with your child's teacher, but you don't know how to get started. Am I hearing you correctly?"
Providing emotional validation	Clinician provides social support, emotional reassurance, and validation of parents' feelings.	"I can see how much you want a plan in place for your child in school, and it's frustrating that it's taking so much time to get things in place."
Building connections among parents	Clinician fosters connections among parents and encourages sharing and problem solving among them.	"I see other heads nodding in response to that last comment. Have others experienced something similar?"
Maintaining parents' focus on FSS principles and intervention components	Clinician keeps discussion organized and focused on research-based principles and practices.	"I know it can be frustrating at times to work with the school. How does criticizing the teacher help your child? What are other ways to address the situation?"

Note. Dimensions developed for the Bootcamp for ADHD program applied for implementation of the FSS program. For additional reading, refer to Fogler and colleagues (2020) and Nissley-Tsiopinis and colleagues (2023).

Encouraging Active Parent Engagement

This dimension refers to clinician efforts to promote parent self-discovery and facilitate the active involvement of each parent in the program. A clinician who facilitates a session with a high level of process fidelity asks key open-ended questions, affirms parents for their participation, makes reflective statements that guide parents in a process of self-discovery, adapts material to individual family situations, and makes a concerted effort to involve each parent.

Eliciting and Strengthening Change Talk

This dimension is based on research that motivational interviewing is effective in promoting behavioral change (Miller & Rollnick, 2023). This dimension refers to the extent to which the provider elicits statements from parents indicating some willingness to change, or at least a willingness to question the status quo (change talk) and provides reinforcement for these statements when they are made. A clinician who is high on this dimension prompts change talk by highlighting statements indicating movement in the direction of change and pointing out discrepancies between statements suggesting a willingness to consider change and behaviors that align with the status quo.

Providing Emotional Validation

This dimension refers to how the clinician responds to expressions of emotion by parents. A clinician who is high on this dimension acknowledges and joins with parents when they express their feelings about a situation; the clinician provides support, emotional reassurance, and validation of the parent's feelings. Even if the parent expresses feelings the clinician does not want to foster (e.g., impatience with the teacher), the clinician expresses empathy and conveys the legitimacy of the parent's feeling.

Building Connections among Parents

This dimension refers to the effectiveness of clinicians in fostering connections among parents and creating a group context that is supportive. Such a context promotes self-empowerment and self-discovery among parents. The clinician who is high on this dimension uses strategies to facilitate interaction among parents (e.g., asking parents to share their reactions to comments made by another parent) and reinforces parents for sharing with and supporting one another. The clinician works to counter the tendency for parents to engage in back-and-forth conversation with the clinician.

Maintaining Parents' Focus on FSS Principles and Intervention Components

This dimension refers to clinician efforts to keep the focus of the discussion on foundational principles and evidence-based practices. At times, discussions in groups can become disorganized or emphasize points that are not consistent with research-based principles and practices. Clinicians who are highly rated on this dimension are consistently strong in keeping the group focused and on task and ensuring group discussions are grounded in sound theory and evidence-based practice. It can be challenging for clinicians to consistently provide emotional validation and promote parent engagement while working to keep the group focused on strategies that work.

For each of the five process fidelity items, raters are asked to distinguish whether clinician actions reflect high or low fidelity. Examples of high and low fidelity are indicated on the *Process Fidelity Checklist* form (see Appendix B). Subsequently raters are requested to indicate whether indications of high (or low) fidelity are sort of true or very true for each dimension. Each fidelity dimension is scored on a scale ranging from 1 = low fidelity to 4 = high fidelity. It is often helpful to rate process fidelity twice for each session—once for the homework review portion of the session and again for the rest of the session when new material is being discussed. The total process fidelity score for each item is the average score for the session. Because the five process fidelity items reflect unique dimensions of intervention implementation, we typically recommend that process fidelity be reported separately by item, although item scores can be combined to form a composite score for process fidelity.

Family Engagement

Session Attendance

A useful, efficient method of examining family engagement in FSS is to record session attendance. Family attendance at psychosocial intervention sessions generally has been shown to be associated with favorable outcomes (Baydar et al., 2003). That being said, other indicators of parental engagement, specifically parental adherence to requests to practice parenting strategies between sessions, have been shown to be more strongly associated with improvements in parenting practices and child outcomes (Clarke et al., 2015; Nix et al., 2009).

Parental Adherence: Completion of Between-Session Homework Assignments

Parent adherence to requests to practice FSS strategies at home between sessions can be assessed by coding the extent to which between-session homework assignments are completed. Based on the coding system our team developed, each worksheet is scored as follows: 0 = not attempted at all or missing; 1 = attempted but not completed; 2 = completed. The total score across worksheets reflects overall level of adherence, which has been shown to be associated with improvement in parenting and child outcomes (Clarke et al., 2015; Morris et al., 2019). Our research has shown that homework samples can be scored according to established criteria with high levels of interrater agreement ($M = 92.2\%$; Clarke et al., 2015). The coding manual for scoring each homework assignment is in Appendix C.

Parental adherence to between-session homework assignments can also be assessed by requesting FSS providers respond to the following item after each session: "Please rate how well the parent implemented the homework assignment." Clinicians respond to this item using a 7-point Likert scale ranging from 1 = not at all to 7 = a great deal. Clinicians are asked to rate this item based on all available information, including completed homework assignments and/or parent report during the homework review section of each FSS session. This rating is especially important when clinicians have difficulty collecting completed homework from parents, such as when delivering sessions using telehealth. Research has shown that clinician ratings of adherence are associated with child outcomes in response to psychosocial interventions for children with ADHD (Rooney et al., 2018).

MEASURES OF FAMILY AND FAMILY–SCHOOL RELATIONSHIP OUTCOMES

The FSS program directly targets parenting practices, quality of the family–school relationship, and family involvement in education. The following measures have been used to assess these outcome variables.

- *Parent–Child Relationship Questionnaire (PCRQ).* The PCRQ (Furman & Giberson, 1995) *assesses parent perceptions of their parenting practices.* Two factors have been highly useful in examining outcomes for the FSS program: negative/ineffective discipline and positive parenting (Booster et al., 2016; Clarke et al., 2015; Mautone et al., 2012; Power et al., 2012). With permission from the developer, our team has updated this measure for outcome assessment.

The adapted version used for this program comprises 11 items referring to negative/ineffective discipline and 3 items related to positive parenting. Parents respond to items by indicating how frequently they employ each parenting practice using a 5-point Likert scale ranging from 1 = hardly at all to 5 = extremely much. The validity of this scale has been supported in research conducted by Hinshaw and colleagues (2000). This measure is included in Appendix C.

- *Parent–Teacher Involvement Questionnaire (PTIQ).* The PTIQ (Kohl et al., 2000) was developed to assist in evaluating outcomes for the FAST Track study. This measure is firmly rooted in theory and empirical research related to family–school relationships. A unique contribution of this scale is that it *assesses the quality of the family–school relationship* from the perspective of both parents and teachers. This measure includes six parent-report items and five teacher-report items, each rated on a 5-point Likert scale. Internal consistency has been shown to be high for the parent-reported scale (alpha = .90) and teacher-rated scale (alpha = .84; Mautone et al., 2015). See *https://fasttrackproject.org/measure/parent-teacher-involvement-parent/*.

- *Parent as Educator Scale (PES).* The PES (Hoover-Dempsey et al., 1992) is a 10-item scale of family involvement in education, *assessing parent views of their competence in assisting with their children's education.* Parents indicate their agreement with each statement on a 5-point Likert scale ranging from 1 = strongly disagree to 5 = strongly agree. The alpha coefficient for this scale among families of children with ADHD has been shown to be acceptable (Power et al., 2012).

MEASURES OF CHILD OUTCOMES

The following measures may be useful in examining outcomes at the level of the child. These outcomes are more distal than family outcomes because the mechanism of action of the FSS program is to work primarily through parents and teachers to achieve change at the level of the child. We do not recommend administering all of these measures with parents and/or teachers, as doing so would likely be burdensome.

Child Functioning at Home: Parent-Report Child Outcome Measures

- *Behavioral Health Checklist (BHCL).* The BHCL (Power, Koshy, et al., 2013) includes two sections: (1) 18 items *assessing internalizing, externalizing, and ADHD symptoms* (i.e., psychopathology section) and (2) 9 items *assessing social relationships and emotion regulation* (i.e., strength-based section). Separate versions were created (for ages 4–7 and 8–12) to account for developmental variations. To reduce the burden on parents, users might consider administering only four items from the strength-based factor (i.e., has self-control, relates well with teachers, gets along with peers, and relates well with parents). This measure yields separate scores for internalizing, externalizing, ADHD, and strengths.

All items are rated on a scale from 1 = never or rarely to 4 = very often. The factor structure of the BHCL psychopathology section of both versions has been supported for the total sample, as well as demographic subgroups (assigned sex, age, race, ethnicity, and income level; Power, Koshy, et al., 2013), and both versions have been shown to have strong predictive validity (Koshy et al., 2016). The validity of the BHCL strength-based section has also been demonstrated, and this factor has been shown to moderate (buffer) the adverse effects of ADHD, externalizing, and internalizing symptoms on children's social functioning (Mautone et al., 2020). This measure is included in Appendix C.

- *Homework Performance Questionnaire—Parent Version (HPQ-P).* The HPQ-P (Power et al., 2015) is a parent-rated measure of homework that includes 4 items assessing *homework context* and 16 items *assessing student self-regulation* (i.e., productivity, efficiency, organization) *and competence* (i.e., ability to understand homework and complete work independently). Each item is rated on a 4-point scale (ranging from 0 = rarely/never to 3 = always/almost always) to reflect the frequency with which each behavior occurs. The measure yields a total score as well as subscale scores for self-regulation and competence. Research supports the internal consistency and validity of this measure (Power et al., 2015). This measure is available in English and Spanish and both versions are included in Appendix C.

- *Homework Problem Checklist (HPC).* The HPC (Anesko et al., 1987) is a measure *assessing parents' perceptions of their child's homework performance*. Each item is rated on a 4-point scale with 0 = never and 3 = very often, indicating how frequently the child manifests common homework problems. The HPC yields a total score and two factor scores: avoidance/inefficiency (e.g., child puts off doing work and child daydreams) and organization/materials management (e.g., child does not know assignments and child does not return assignments to class; Langberg et al., 2010; Power et al., 2006). A substantial body of research supports the use of the HPC as an outcome measure for psychosocial interventions targeting children with ADHD (Abikoff et al., 2013; Langberg et al., 2018; Power et al., 2012).

- *Impairment Rating Scale—Parent Version (IRS-P).* The IRS (Fabiano et al., 2006) *examines areas of functioning known to be impaired in children with ADHD*. The parent version includes six domains (relationship with peers, relationship with parents, academic progress, self-esteem, influence on family functioning, and overall severity of the problem). An item related to siblings can also be included, but it may not be relevant for all families. Raters are asked to indicate the degree to which the child's problems have affected functioning in a specific area during the past 2 weeks on a 6-point Likert scale ranging from 0 (no problem/definitely does not need treatment or special services) to 6 (extreme problem/definitely needs treatment or special services). The IRS-P has been found to correlate with informant ratings of similar domains of impairment using other measures and observations of classroom and nonclassroom behavior in a summer treatment camp (Fabiano et al., 2006).

Child Functioning at School: Teacher-Report Child Outcome Measures

- *Homework Performance Questionnaire—Teacher Version (HPQ-T).* The HPQ-T (Power at al., 2015) is a teacher-rated measure of homework that includes 8 items assessing the *context of homework* and 23 items *assessing student self-regulation and competence in completing homework*. Each item is rated on a 7-point scale to reflect the percentage of time that each behavior occurs (0 = 0–10%; 6 = 91–100%). The HPQ-T yields a total score as well as subscale scores for self-regulation (i.e., productivity, organization, efficiency) and competence (i.e., ability to understand homework and complete work independently). Research supports the internal consistency as well as validity of this measure in a general sample of students (Power et al., 2015). This measure is included in Appendix C.

- *Impairment Rating Scale—Teacher Version (IRS-T).* The teacher version of the IRS *assesses areas of functioning known to be impacted by ADHD*. This measure contains six domains (relationship with peers, relationship with teacher, academic progress, self-esteem, influence on classroom functioning, and overall severity of the problem; Fabiano et al., 2006). Raters are asked to indicate the degree to which the child's problems have affected functioning in a specific area during the past 2 weeks on a 6-point Likert scale ranging from 0 (no problem/definitely does not need treatment or special services) to 6 (extreme problem/definitely needs treatment or special services). As indicated above, substantial research supports the validity of the IRS (Fabiano et al., 2006).

- *Academic Proficiency Scale (APS).* The APS (Abikoff et al., 2013) is a teacher-report measure that *assesses proficiency in six academic subjects* (reading, spelling, language arts, social studies, science, and math) relative to standard expectations (0 = well below standard expected at this time of year; 2 = at standard; 4 = well above standard). The total mean item score is the unit of analysis. The reliability of this scale has been shown to be acceptable (alpha = .84; Abikoff et al., 2013). The APS is recommended instead of obtaining student report card grades because grading systems vary substantially across schools and the timing of report cards often does not align with outcome assessment periods. This measure is included in Appendix C.

MEASURE OF PROGRAM SATISFACTION

- *FSS Program Evaluation Scale.* Our team has developed a FSS Program Evaluation Scale to *assess parents' satisfaction with the FSS program*. There are four parts to the scale: (1) evaluation of major components of the program (e.g., Child's Game, antecedent–behavior–consequence model, homework strategies; items 1–6); (2) evaluation of intervention procedures (e.g., handouts, phone calls to parents, between-session homework assignments; items 7–11); (3) evaluation of clinician effectiveness (e.g., good job managing time; respectful of family; understanding of family situation; items 12–17); and (4) comments about what was most helpful and what could make the intervention more effective in the future. Participants respond to items 1 to 11 using a 4-point Likert scale: 1 = not very helpful to 4 = very helpful; and they respond to items 12–17 using a 4-point scale ranging from 1 = disagree to 4 = agree. Given that this form collects information that is sensitive in nature and should be kept private, in particular data about clinician effectiveness, we recommend that parents complete the forms anonymously. It should be acknowledged that it may be challenging to protect privacy when FSS is provided in groups of three or fewer families. When there are only a small number of families participating, it may be advisable to omit items related to clinician effectiveness. We also suggest that clinicians give consent to having this information collected and understand how the information will be used. This measure is included in Appendix C.

CONCLUSIONS

This chapter describes a plan for FSS program evaluation that is aligned with the theory of change described in Chapter 2. The plan includes methods for evaluating child outcomes, potential mechanisms of action (i.e., parenting practices, quality of the family–school relationship), clinician fidelity of implementation, participant engagement, and program satisfaction. Although we strongly recommend the incorporation of program evaluation strategies when implementing FSS, the plan that actually gets implemented will depend on whether the program is being offered in a research or clinical context. In addition, when evaluating outcomes in clinical practice, it is important to consider the time it takes to administer and score measures and what will be acceptable to participating families.

CHAPTER 16

Assessing the Outcomes of Family–School Success

with Yael Gross and Katie Tremont

This chapter describes the intervention outcomes of families who participated in two FSS groups that were offered in the context of a hospital-based ADHD center. These cases are presented to describe the range of outcomes that can occur in response to this intervention. It should be noted that the evaluation of outcomes for these cases was conducted in the context of routine clinical practice, not in the context of a rigorous, randomized controlled trial (RCT). For a description of outcomes of FSS examined in the context of a RCT, see Chapter 2. The reader is also referred to studies published by Power and colleagues (2012) and Mautone and colleagues (2012). This chapter provides a description of how FSS was implemented with two groups of families and includes the following sections:

- Context of FSS program implementation
- Program participants and intervention procedures
- Outcome measures administered
- Results: Program satisfaction
- Results: Intervention outcomes

Yael Gross, MA, is a doctoral student in the School Psychology Program at Lehigh University in Pennsylvania and contributed to this chapter as a clinical research coordinator at Children's Hospital of Philadelphia.

Katie Tremont, MPH, obtained her master's degree in public health from the University of Pennsylvania in 2016. She has managed large federally funded clinical trials in the behavioral sciences as a project manager at CHOP.

CONTEXT OF FSS PROGRAM IMPLEMENTATION

The two FSS groups described in this chapter were conducted in the winter of 2021–2022, approximately 2 years after the COVID-19 pandemic began in March 2020. Groups were interrupted by the school break during the winter holidays. At the time of intervention and data collection, there was a spike in COVID-19 cases in our region due primarily to the Omicron variant. During this time, families were continuing to experience heightened stress due to the pandemic (Adams et al., 2021). Schools generally were educating students in the classroom, but most schools in the region were continuing to impose mask mandates on students and staff. The level of stress among educators was high (Kotowski et al., 2022), and there were elevated rates of student and staff absenteeism.

In this context, these two FSS groups were provided to families via telehealth. Group sessions were conducted in the early evening (starting between 5:00 and 5:30 P.M.) and lasted approximately 75 minutes. Children were expected to attend each session for at least 30 minutes. The purposes of involving children in the sessions were to orient them to FSS strategies, give parents and children an opportunity to learn and practice strategies together, and enable clinicians to meet requirements to bill for multifamily group therapy.

To collect outcome data for the purpose of reporting findings in presentations and publications, data collection was conducted in the context of a research study approved by the Institutional Review Board of the hospital. All families invited to participate in the study were informed that providing outcome data was optional and not required to participate in the FSS group. For group 1, four families were approached to participate and three enrolled. For group 2, five families were approached to participate, and all five families enrolled. However, in group 2, one of the five families did not complete any questionnaires, and a second family did not provide any posttreatment or follow-up data. As such, this chapter reports outcomes for three families in group 1 and three families in group 2. Families received a stipend for completing measures at each timepoint and they were informed that they would receive a report of outcome findings after their participation in the study.

PROGRAM PARTICIPANTS AND INTERVENTION PROCEDURES

Families were initially referred to the FSS program based in the ADHD center by clinicians practicing in a tertiary care children's hospital in a large metropolitan area. Although a diagnosis of ADHD was not required for participation, all of the children described in this chapter had been diagnosed with ADHD. In addition, two of the children met criteria for oppositional defiant disorder and one was assessed as having a global developmental delay. Children in the two groups were ages 6–9.

The two groups described in this chapter were conducted by different clinicians. Each of the clinicians was a psychologist practicing in the ADHD center with at least 5 years of experience. For the first group, three trainees (i.e., two psychology interns and a child psychiatry fellow) in addition to the psychologist were involved in delivering the FSS program. Trainees co-led sessions, periodically conducted phone calls with families throughout the program, and attempted to reach out to children's teachers to support family–school collaboration and classroom-based intervention development. There were no trainees involved in the second group. The psychologist for the second group was not able to make phone calls to families or teachers during the program. For both groups, the FSS program was provided in a total of eight sessions. The curriculum for Sessions 6 and 7 (focused on behavioral homework interventions) was combined into one session in order to reduce the length of the program to eight sessions.

OUTCOME MEASURES ADMINISTERED

Outcome measures included five scales administered to parents at baseline, posttreatment, and follow-up 3 months after the end of intervention: the Parent–Child Relationship Questionnaire (PCRQ), the Parent–Teacher Involvement Questionnaire, Quality of the Parent–Teacher Relationship subscale (PTIQ; parent version), the Impairment Rating Scale (IRS; parent version), the Homework Performance Questionnaire (HPQ; parent version), and the Behavioral Health Checklist (BHCL). (See Chapter 15 for information about these measures.) Parent measures were collected by emailing parents a link to complete an electronic survey through the Research Electronic Data Capture (REDCap) system (Harris et al., 2009) hosted at our institution. We attempted to collect outcome data from teachers for two children but did not receive a response to email inquiries and hence were unable to collect school data. We stopped contacting school personnel after being offered advice by numerous colleagues working in education that continuing to pursue these data would impose an undue burden on teachers due to the COVID-19 pandemic. For brevity, the tables in this chapter report findings from outcome measures that were most sensitive to change in response to FSS. In addition to the five parental outcome measures, we collected data about family attendance at sessions and parent completion of between-session homework assignments, which were scored using the manual included in Appendix C.

RESULTS

Program Satisfaction

Five parents completed the Family–School Success Program Evaluation Scale. This questionnaire has three sections: (1) perception of program content, (2) perception of implementation supports, and (3) perception of clinician effectiveness. Perception of both program content (e.g., topics for discussion) and implementation supports (e.g., handouts, between-session homework assignments) were rated on a 4-point scale (1 = not very helpful; 2 = somewhat helpful; 3 = helpful; 4 = very helpful). Perception of clinician effectiveness was also rated on a 4-point scale (1 = disagree; 2 = somewhat disagree; 3 = somewhat agree; 4 = agree). Ratings of program content varied from a mean item score of 3.0 to 3.6. Higher ratings (3.6) were reported for content strategies focused on improving child homework and school performance. Lower ratings (3.0–3.2), still in the favorable range, were reported for content strategies focused on caregiver self-care and the use of punishment. Ratings of implementation supports demonstrated more variability. Higher ratings (3.2–3.4) were reported for the helpfulness of program handouts, between-session homework assignments, and the opportunity to share with other parents. A relatively low rating (2.6) was assigned for telephone contacts with the school, reflecting differences between groups in both clinician ability to reach out to teachers and clinician ability to connect with teachers. On the third section of the questionnaire, parents assigned high ratings to items reflecting perceptions of clinician effectiveness (3.4–4.0), indicating parents had favorable views about the organization of sessions and the respectfulness of interactions with clinicians. This scale is included in Appendix C.

Feedback shared by parents in comments at the end of the questionnaire indicated they appreciated the opportunity to share their experiences with other parents and gain knowledge and skills through participation in the program. Two parents raised questions about the helpfulness of involving children in the sessions and suggested that clinicians provide more guidance about how to make sessions meaningful for children.

Intervention Outcomes

The outcomes for families consenting to participate in the program evaluation study are reported in Table 16.1. Criteria for determining whether the improvement from preintervention to postintervention and follow-up was meaningful are indicated in the table note. As indicated, average session attendance across the six families was 85% (ranging from 75% to 100%). As expected, all parents demonstrated movement in the expected direction on the PCRQ at postintervention and/or follow-up, and three of the six parents demonstrated a meaningful reduction in negative parenting at postintervention and/or follow-up. Four children demonstrated a meaningful reduction in level of impairment (IRS; parent version) at postintervention and/or follow-up, and in two cases the reduction was meaningful and large. All children demonstrated movement in the expected direction on the HPQ and in two cases child improvement in homework performance was meaningful at follow-up. In addition, three of six parents reported a meaningful increase in child strengths (BHCL) at postintervention and/or follow-up.

Consistent with prior research on the positive association between family engagement in FSS and intervention outcomes (Clarke et al., 2015), the family with the most favorable outcomes (see Child 1, Table 16.1) attended all sessions and completed all between-session homework assignments. It should be noted that the family of Child 3 reported a substantial amount of family stress during the intervention and also reported experiencing a major family disruption near the end of the intervention. In this family, negative parenting increased and the quality of the parent–teacher relationship decreased from preintervention to postintervention. However, there was substantial movement in the expected direction on both of these outcomes at the time of follow-up.

After intervention, three of the six families expressed interest in a referral for additional intervention, including individualized behavioral therapy (Child 2, Child 6) and medication (Child 2, Child 3). Reports summarizing the outcome data were sent to parents after the completion of follow-up measures. At the end of this chapter, we have included an example of a report prepared for the parents of Child 6 (*FSS Program Report of Progress*), which illustrates how program findings might be communicated to families participating in the FSS program. Appendix A includes a template handout for creating this report.

Although clinicians commonly include a summary of any available teacher ratings in evaluation reports shared with parents, we recommend that clinicians inform parents and teachers before intervention that teacher ratings will be used to examine outcomes and outcome data based on both parent and teacher ratings will be shared with parents. Parents can choose whether to share the summary with the child's school.

TABLE 16.1. Attendance Rates, Adherence Rates, and Intervention Outcomes for Families in Groups 1 and 2

Child	Child age	Attendance rate	Parent homework completion rate	PCRQ Negative Parenting	PTIQ Parent–Teacher Relationship	IRS Child Impairment	HPQ Child Homework Performance	BHCL Child Strengths
Results of FSS Cohort 1								
Child 1	6 years							
Pre				3.36	1.17	4.50	2.19	8%
Post		100%	100%	2.91	1.50	3.50**	2.31	5%
FU				2.09**	2.33**	3.00**	2.63	13%
Child 2	6 years							
Pre				2.91	0.83	4.00	2.38	20%
Post		75%	57%	3.64	1.33*	5.83	2.69	13%
FU				2.27*	0.50	4.67	2.75	5%
Child 3	9 years							
Pre				3.55	1.50	4.50	1.75	22%
Post		75%	43%	3.91	1.33	4.83	2.13	42%*
FU				3.18	1.67	4.00*	2.25*	32%
Results of FSS Cohort 2								
Child 4	6 years							
Pre				2.36	3.17	3.33	2.00	60%
Post		88%	38%	2.27	3.17	3.67	2.25	35%
FU				2.27	2.50	2.83*	2.56*	60%
Child 5	6 years							
Pre				3.55	2.50	3.67	—	5%
Post		88%	14%	2.73*	2.33	4.67	—	5%
FU				2.64*	2.83	3.50	—	24%*
Child 6	8 years							
Pre				2.64	2.50	3.50	2.56	24%
Post		88%	43%	2.27	2.50	2.33**	2.06	35%
FU				2.45	2.67	2.50**	2.69	47%*

Note. PCRQ, Parent–Child Relationship Questionnaire; PTIQ, Parent–Teacher Involvement Questionnaire; IRS, Impairment Rating Scale; HPQ, Homework Performance Questionnaire; BHCL, Behavioral Health Checklist; Pre, preintervention; Post, postintervention; FU, follow-up 3 months after postintervention. Higher scores on the PCRQ Negative Parenting factor reflect more negative parenting. A reduction of ≥ 0.5 is considered meaningful. Higher scores on the PTIQ reflect a more positive parent–teacher relationship. An improvement of ≥ 0.5 is considered meaningful. Higher scores on the IRS reflect greater impairment. A reduction of ≥ 0.5 is considered meaningful. Higher scores on the HPQ reflect better homework performance. An improvement ≥ 0.5 is considered meaningful. Higher scores on the BHCL Strengths factor reflect stronger relationships and better self-regulation. An improvement $\geq 15\%$ is considered meaningful.
* Meaningful improvement in expected direction.
** Meaningful and large improvement in expected direction.

CONCLUSIONS

This chapter illustrates findings that may be obtained when conducting an evaluation of the FSS program. As indicated in Table 16.1, a considerable range of results for family engagement, child outcomes, and potential mechanisms of action can be expected across participants for each FSS cohort. The FSS program was offered to these cohorts at a particularly challenging time (i.e., during an upsurge of the COVID-19 pandemic), which may have exacerbated family stress and posed challenges to parents in working with teachers to strengthen the family–school relationship. Further, it was not possible to collect teacher-report outcome data. Nonetheless, variation in outcomes across measures and participants is quite typical and can be expected when conducting a program evaluation.

It is quite common for families to need additional support and intervention after the program is over. After intervention we routinely recommend that parents involve themselves in parent support groups, such as Children and Adults with Attention-Deficit/Hyperactivity Disorder (CHADD; *www.chadd.org*), to help them sustain gains and address new challenges as these arise. In addition, some families will benefit from follow-up, individualized family behavioral therapy and/or initiation or adjustments of medication after the program ends. Moreover, given that ADHD is a chronic condition, virtually all families will need to reengage in psychosocial interventions at various times during their child's development, particularly during periods of transition (e.g., transition to middle school and high school). As such, families need frequent reminders that the process of intervention is continuous. Families need ongoing support from other families, primary care clinicians, and school professionals, and at times more intensive psychosocial intervention is required.

Family–School Success (FSS) Program Report of Progress

Name of Child: *Child 6*

Date of Birth of Child:

Informant: Mother

Date of Report:

This report describes outcomes for your child and family in response to your recent participation in the Family–School Success program. This program is a multifamily group intervention that includes standard elements of behavioral parent training in addition to behavioral homework interventions, and a classroom behavioral intervention (daily report card). This program was delivered to your family in eight sessions and was provided by telehealth. The following sections describe your child's progress in the program assessed by several measures given preintervention, postintervention, and follow-up (3 months after intervention ended). It was noted that your family attended seven of the eight sessions scheduled.

Domain assessed: Parent–Child Relationship

Measure administered: Parent–Child Relationship Questionnaire (PCRQ). This measure includes two scales assessing parent perceptions of their parenting practices. One scale assesses negative/ineffective parenting and the other scale assesses positive parenting. Scores can be converted to a summary score (ranging from 1 to 5). Lower scores for negative/ineffective parenting are better and indicate less negative parenting. Higher scores for positive parenting are better and indicate more positive parenting. A change in score of 0.5 of a point is considered meaningful.

Negative/Ineffective Parenting

Assessment period	Mean item score
Preintervention	2.64
Postintervention	2.27
Follow-up	2.45

Positive Parenting

Assessment period	Mean item score
Preintervention	4.50
Postintervention	4.00
Follow-up	4.50

Interpretation: Scores indicate there may have been a small reduction in negative parenting from preintervention to postintervention and follow-up, but the degree of change was below the level considered to be meaningful. There was essentially no change in positive parenting, which was already high at preintervention.

Domain assessed: Quality of the Parent–Teacher Relationship

Measure administered: Parent–Teacher Involvement Questionnaire (PTIQ). This measure is used to assess the parent–teacher relationship from the parent perspective. The measure yields a summary score (ranging from 0 to 4), with higher ratings indicating a better parent–teacher relationship. A change of 0.5 of a point is considered meaningful.

Quality of the Parent–Teacher Relationship

Assessment period	Mean item score
Preintervention	2.50
Postintervention	2.50
Follow-up	2.67

Interpretation: There was no change in ratings of the family–school relationship after FSS or at follow-up.

Domains assessed: ADHD Symptoms, Anxiety/Depression, Disruptive Behavior

Measure administered: Behavioral Health Checklist (BHCL). The first section of this scale assesses child ADHD symptoms, anxiety/depression, and disruptive behaviors. The second section assesses child strengths in interpersonal relationships. Scores on these scales are converted to percentile scores. Lower percentile scores for ADHD symptoms, anxiety/depression, and disruptive behaviors indicate fewer problems. Higher percentiles on the child's strengths domain indicate more strengths. A change of 15 percentile points is considered meaningful.

ADHD Symptoms

Assessment period	Percentile
Preintervention	>99th
Postintervention	94th
Follow-up	69th

Anxiety/Depression Symptoms

Assessment period	Percentile
Preintervention	83rd
Postintervention	89th–90th
Follow-up	92nd–93rd

Disruptive Behaviors

Assessment period	Percentile
Preintervention	70th
Postintervention	46th–47th
Follow-up	46th–47th

Child Strengths

Assessment period	Percentile
Preintervention	23rd–24th
Postintervention	35th
Follow-up	47th

Interpretation: Ratings show a meaningful reduction in child ADHD symptoms and disruptive behaviors at the time of postintervention and/or follow-up and a meaningful increase in report of child strengths at follow-up. There was essentially no change in ratings of child anxiety and depression.

Domains assessed: Child Impairment in Academic and Interpersonal Functioning

Measure administered: Impairment Rating Scale (IRS). This parent-report measure assesses whether a child is experiencing problems in several domains of functioning, including relationships with peers, relationships with parents, academic performance, self-esteem, and family functioning. This measure yields a summary score (ranging from 0 to 6) with lower scores indicating less overall impairment. A change of 0.5 point is considered meaningful.

Child Impairment

Assessment period	Mean item score
Preintervention	3.50
Postintervention	2.33
Follow-up	2.50

Interpretation: Overall, ratings on this measure indicate a large reduction in impairment when comparing preintervention with postintervention and follow-up.

Domain assessed: Homework Performance

Measure administered: Homework Performance Questionnaire—Parent Version (HPQ-P). This parent-report measure assesses a range of child homework behaviors, including a set of behaviors related to homework productivity, time management, and organization of materials. This scale can be converted to a summary score (ranging from 0 to 3), with higher scores indicating better homework performance. An increase of 0.5 point is considered meaningful.

Homework Performance

Assessment period	Mean item score
Preintervention	2.56
Postintervention	2.06
Follow-up	2.69

Interpretation: There was a meaningful movement in the unexpected direction (i.e., reduction in homework performance) at postintervention but a return to essentially baseline level at follow-up.

Overall Summary

Domains in Which There Was Improvement

Lower child ADHD symptoms
Less child disruptive behavior
Less overall child impairment

Domains in Which There Was No Change

Parenting practices
Quality of parent–teacher relationship
Child anxiety/depression symptoms
Homework performance

Domains in Which There Was a Decline

None

Recommendations

- The parents/caregivers may wish to share this report with their child's primary care clinician as well as school staff.
- The parents/caregivers are strongly encouraged to continue using the strategies discussed in the Family–School Success program. In particular, each family developed a formula for success, indicating the strategies that were most useful in helping their child with challenges at home and school. Parents/caregivers are strongly advised to reflect on their formula for success and implement the strategies that are most useful to them on a consistent basis.

APPENDIX A

Parent Handouts and Homework Assignments

Note: Only the initial reference of each handout is listed; some handouts are used in more than one session.

SESSION 1

Handout—Welcome to Family–School Success	155
Handout—Program Schedule	157
Handout—FSS "Big Ideas"	158
Handout—Family–School Success Theory of Change	159
Handout—Attention-Deficit/Hyperactivity Disorder (ADHD)—Basic Facts	160
Handout—Attention Grid: Adult Attention as a Consequence	164
Handout—Catch Them Being Good	165
Handout—Homework—Noticing Positive/Desired Behavior	167

SESSION 2

Handout—Child's Game	168
Handout—Homework—Child's Game	170

SESSION 3

Handout—The A-B-C Model of Behavior	171
Handout—Effective Instructions	172
Handout—Understanding and Changing the Consequences of Behavior	173
Handout—Using Positive Reinforcement	175
Handout—Homework—A-B-C Worksheet	179
Handout—Homework—Reward Menu	180

SESSION 4

Handout—Tips for Building Partnerships with Teachers	181
Handout—Developing a Daily Report Card	182
Handout—Sample Daily Report Card—NOT RECOMMENDED	183
Handout—Sample Daily Report Card 1	184
Handout—Sample Daily Report Card 2	185

SESSION 5

Handout—Establishing a Token Economy	186
Handout—Homework—Target Behaviors	189
Handout—Homework—Home Rewards Worksheet	190

SESSION 6

Handout—Establishing the Homework Ritual	191
Handout—Homework—Homework A-B-C Worksheet	193
Handout—Homework—Homework Ritual Worksheet	194

SESSION 7

Handout—Managing Time and Goal Setting	195
Handout—Goal-Setting Tool	197

SESSION 8

Handout—Using Punishment Successfully	198
Handout—Punishment Discussion Questions	199
Handout—Homework—Using Punishment Strategically	200

SESSION 9

Handout—How to Address Challenging Situations	201
Handout—Challenging Situations Worksheet	202
Handout—Maintaining Success and Anticipating Future Problems	203
Handout—Formula for Success	206
Handout—Finding a Provider for Behavior Management with ADHD	208
Handout—Certificate of Completion	210
Handout—Template for Report of Progress	211

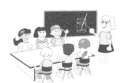

FAMILY–SCHOOL SUCCESS

SESSION 1

Welcome to Family–School Success

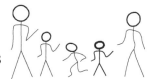

We welcome you and your child to the Family–School Success program. This program is designed to assist your family in promoting your child's success at home and school and in developing a more satisfying and positive parent–child relationship.

Our Approach

We use what is called a *behavioral approach* in this program. This means we focus on identifying and targeting environmental influences on a child's actions. Specifically, we are interested in examining and changing the events that occur before and after a problem behavior and that may serve to evoke or maintain a problem. **The key to a behavioral approach is to focus on events that can be changed and not to focus on characteristics that are very difficult to change.**

Please bring a binder or folder to each session, as we will be distributing worksheets and educational handouts each week. For the first few weeks, we request that you wear your name tag. In order to get the most out of the program, we also ask that you follow these guidelines:

1. **Please arrive at each session on time.** We will meet on the same evening each week for 90 minutes.

2. **Participate!** By expressing your concerns and voicing your opinions, you will gain much support from one another and will have a greater opportunity to learn and to address the needs of your family.

3. **Listen!** In this group, you will discover that you are not alone. Parents repeatedly tell us how much they have benefited from listening to the experiences of others as to how they deal with the problems faced during homework time.

4. **Do your homework.** This is an active, goal-directed program. Parents who are committed to improving their child's behavior consistently do their Family–School Success assignments. One way to ensure that you do not become overly frustrated is to allow us to assist you in troubleshooting problems with assignments.

5. **Communicate with your child's teacher.** Frequent and collaborative home–school communication is essential to achieve the goals of this program. Ask questions of your child's teacher and be sure to let them know how your child is progressing on Family–School Success goals.

6. **Contact us.** Do not hesitate to call or message us if you experience problems when doing your between-session assignments during the week.

7. **Respect confidentiality.** A key requirement of Family–School Success is that you not discuss other families' problems and issues outside of the session room.

(continued)

Adapted from Power, Karustis, and Habboushe (2001). Copyright © 2001 The Guilford Press. Reprinted by permission in *Family–School Success for Children with ADHD: A Guide for Intervention* by Thomas J. Power, Jennifer A. Mautone, and Stephen L. Soffer (The Guilford Press, 2024). Permission to photocopy this material, or to download and print additional copies (*www.guilford.com/power2-forms*), is granted to purchasers of this book for personal use or use with students; see copyright page for details.

Welcome to Family–School Success *(page 2 of 2)*

8. **Hang in there.** Although many families begin to experience positive effects from the program right away, benefits will usually tend to become more evident as the group unfolds. We encourage you and your child to work hard and try to remain patient—hang in there.

9. **Be hopeful!** Addressing difficulties at home and school is a very challenging process. However, we are confident that if you consistently attend, listen, actively participate, and work very hard to apply these strategies, you will observe some very positive changes in your child's behavior, as well as in your relationship with your child.

10. **Try to enjoy the process!** Strange as this may sound while you and your child are experiencing behavior problems and conflicts, the process of working on improving home and school performance does not have to be painful. We strongly encourage you to take note of the gains that you make and to celebrate them.

FAMILY–SCHOOL SUCCESS
SESSION 1
Program Schedule

Date	Time	Location	Topic
			Session 1: Introducing Family–School Success
			Session 2: Strengthening Family Relationships
			Session 3: Understanding the Basics of Behavior Management
			Session 4: Preparing for Family–School Collaboration
			Session 5: Introducing the Token Economy
			Session 6: Understanding the Function of Behavior and Establishing the Homework Ritual
			Session 7: Managing Time and Goal Setting
			Session 8: Using Punishment Successfully
			Session 9: Planning for Future Success

From *Family–School Success for Children with ADHD: A Guide for Intervention* by Thomas J. Power, Jennifer A. Mautone, and Stephen L. Soffer. Copyright © 2024 The Guilford Press. Permission to photocopy this material, or to download and print additional copies (*www.guilford.com/power2-forms*), is granted to purchasers of this book for personal use or use with students; see copyright page for details.

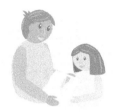

FAMILY–SCHOOL SUCCESS
SESSION 1
FSS "Big Ideas"

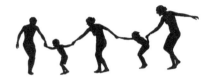

Throughout the program, we will refer to "big ideas," or important principles, that form the foundation for Family–School Success. Remember that a major goal of this program is to help families promote their children's educational success. The following ideas are critical for children's development and educational success. As you learn new material each week and as your child grows, keep these "big ideas" in mind.

A strong parent–child relationship is critical for successful child development.

A strong, affirming parent–child relationship enables children to view themselves as valuable and important persons. Ongoing interactions between parents and children help children learn how to manage their behavior and emotions. Children with strong parent–child relationships are prepared for successful relationships with others outside the home and are prepared to manage their behavior and emotions in challenging situations at school and in the community.

A home environment that supports learning promotes school success.

Family involvement in children's education contributes to school success. Families can be involved in education by participating in school activities, establishing a strong relationship with school professionals, and working to strengthen the family–school relationship throughout the academic year. Families can also be involved in education by creating a home environment that supports learning. For example, families can make education a priority, set aside time for literacy activities, and limit television viewing. Families can also take advantage of natural learning opportunities that exist in the daily routine, such as counting money while shopping and following instructions when baking.

The parent–teacher relationship impacts children's school performance.

Parent–teacher collaboration is important for supporting children's educational performance. When parents and teachers have a strong relationship, they are able to work together effectively to acknowledge and enhance student strengths and provide support at home and school when there are difficulties. In addition, the relationship that parents have with teachers affects the relationship between teachers and students. Just as it is important to develop a strong parent–child relationship, it is important that there is a strong relationship between the teacher and the child. Successful teacher–student relationships contribute to strong academic achievement and effective peer interactions at school.

From *Family–School Success for Children with ADHD: A Guide for Intervention* by Thomas J. Power, Jennifer A. Mautone, and Stephen L. Soffer. Copyright © 2024 The Guilford Press. Permission to photocopy this material, or to download and print additional copies (*www.guilford.com/power2-forms*), is granted to purchasers of this book for personal use or use with students; see copyright page for details.

FAMILY–SCHOOL SUCCESS

SESSION 1

Family–School Success Theory of Change

FSS Goals

- Strengthen Parenting and Parent–Child Relationship
- Strengthen Parent Effectiveness
- Improve Family Involvement in Education and Family–School Collaboration

→ Child Functioning at Home → Child Functioning at School

From *Family–School Success for Children with ADHD: A Guide for Intervention* by Thomas J. Power, Jennifer A. Mautone, and Stephen L. Soffer. Copyright © 2024 The Guilford Press. Permission to photocopy this material, or to download and print additional copies (*www.guilford.com/power2-forms*), is granted to purchasers of this book for personal use or use with students; see copyright page for details.

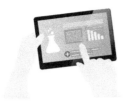
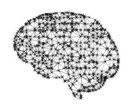

FAMILY–SCHOOL SUCCESS
SESSION 1

Attention-Deficit/Hyperactivity Disorder (ADHD)—Basic Facts

What is ADHD?
- Attention-deficit/hyperactivity disorder (ADHD) is a neurodevelopmental disorder that affects control of behavior, attention, and emotions.
- Core symptoms of ADHD are inattention, impulsivity, and hyperactivity.

How many people have ADHD?
- The mean (average) estimate is approximately 9%.
- There are more males than females—approximately a 2:1 ratio of males to females.

What are the symptoms of ADHD?
- There are two types of ADHD symptoms—inattention and hyperactivity/impulsivity.

  Inattention (9 symptoms):
  o Often fails to give close attention to details
  o Often has difficulty sustaining attention to tasks
  o Often does not listen when spoken to directly
  o Often does not follow through on instructions
  o Often has difficulty organizing tasks
  o Often avoids tasks requiring sustained effort
  o Often loses things necessary for tasks
  o Often easily distracted
  o Often forgetful in daily activities

  Hyperactivity/Impulsivity (9 symptoms):
  o Often fidgets with hands or feet
  o Often leaves seat in classroom or other situations
  o Often runs about excessively
  o Often has difficulty playing quietly
  o Often acts as if "driven by a motor"
  o Often talks excessively
  o Often blurts out answers before questions have been completed
  o Often has difficulty awaiting turn
  o Often interrupts others

What are the additional diagnostic criteria?
- Presence of symptoms for at least 6 months
- At least 6 of 9 symptoms of hyperactivity/impulsivity and/or inattention
- Behaviors inconsistent with developmental level
- Several symptoms of inattention and/or hyperactivity/impulsivity present in multiple settings
- Symptoms contribute to functional impairment (social and/or academic)

(continued)

Adapted from Power, Karustis, and Habboushe (2001). Copyright © 2001 The Guilford Press. Reprinted by permission in *Family–School Success for Children with ADHD: A Guide for Intervention* by Thomas J. Power, Jennifer A. Mautone, and Stephen L. Soffer (The Guilford Press, 2024). Permission to photocopy this material, or to download and print additional copies (*www.guilford.com/power2-forms*), is granted to purchasers of this book for personal use or use with students; see copyright page for details.

Attention-Deficit/Hyperactivity Disorder (ADHD)—Basic Facts (page 2 of 4)

- Symptoms present before age 12
- Symptoms not explained by other disorders (e.g., learning disabilities, anxiety disorders, mood disorders)

There are 3 subtypes or presentations of ADHD.

ADHD presentations are largely determined by the symptoms that are present:

1. **ADHD, Predominantly Hyperactive/Impulsive Presentation** (approximately 10% of those with ADHD)
   - The individual has 6 or more of the hyperactivity/impulsivity symptoms but fewer than 6 inattention symptoms.
2. **ADHD, Predominantly Inattentive Presentation** (approximately 40%)
   - The individual has 6 or more of the inattention symptoms but fewer than 6 hyperactivity/impulsivity symptoms.
3. **ADHD, Combined Presentation** (approximately 50%)
   - The individual has 6 or more of the inattention symptoms <u>and</u> 6 or more of the hyperactivity/impulsivity symptoms.

Do children "grow out of ADHD"?

The severity of hyperactivity tends to decrease when children reach adolescence. However, symptoms of inattention and impulsivity remain relatively stable into adulthood.

- About 50% of children with ADHD continue to meet criteria for ADHD in late adolescence.
  - 80% will retain some ADHD symptoms and demonstrate some impairment.

With effective treatment, most children with ADHD can develop skills to cope with their symptoms, and eventually become successful in important areas of their lives. Given that ADHD is a chronic condition, it is important to continually review intervention plans and modify the type and intensity of interventions as needed.

What are the causes of ADHD?

Let's start with what <u>does not</u> cause ADHD:

- ADHD is not caused by faulty parenting.
- ADHD is not caused by poor teachers.
- ADHD is not caused by junk food.

Most evidence supports that biological factors have the strongest contribution to an individual having ADHD. These include:

- Genetic factors (genetic inheritance is likely the strongest contributing factor)
  - Sibling of child with ADHD has 15–25% chance of having ADHD (higher if sibling is male)
  - Identical twin: 80% chance of ADHD if identical twin has ADHD
  - If there is a child with ADHD, there is about a 33% chance that a biological parent has ADHD
- Low birth weight
- Fetal exposure to alcohol or other substances
- Exposure to lead

We also understand that ADHD is likely an outcome of the interaction of genetic/biological factors and environmental factors, such as:

- Stress and trauma
- Poor attachment with caregivers

(continued)

Attention-Deficit/Hyperactivity Disorder (ADHD)—Basic Facts *(page 3 of 4)*

- Prolonged, significant parent–child conflict
- Ineffective schooling

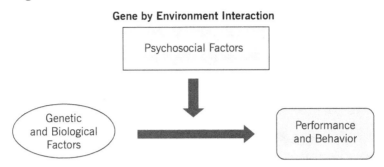

How does ADHD change over the lifespan?

Although ADHD is a chronic condition, the presentation of ADHD may vary as individuals grow from early childhood into adolescence and adulthood.

Preschool years

- Highest levels of hyperactivity, which may result in school dismissal

Elementary school years

- Inattention becomes more salient, resulting in academic problems
- Hyperactivity contributes to disruptive behavior and peer rejection

Middle school years

- Hyperactivity may wane, but impulsivity persists, contributing to peer problems
- Problems with disorganization, time management, and planning become salient

High school and college years

- Inattention and disorganization remain salient, which may have effects on school engagement and performance
- Impulsivity leads to heightened risk taking, which may have harmful effects (drug use, risky driving, risky sexual behavior)
- Youth may have problems transitioning to greater independent functioning, resulting in need for greater adult involvement (importance of mentoring)

Do children with ADHD also have other conditions?

It is common for children with ADHD to have other psychiatric conditions and/or learning difficulties. Individuals with ADHD may have more than one other psychiatric condition. Some common conditions that may be present along with ADHD include (approximate frequency of occurrence with ADHD):

- Learning disabilities (LD; 30%)
- Oppositional defiant disorder (ODD; 40%)
- Conduct disorder (CD; 15%)
- Anxiety disorders (25%)
- Mood disorders (15%, including disruptive mood dysregulation disorder)
- Tic disorders (15%)
- Autism spectrum disorders (10%)

(continued)

Attention-Deficit/Hyperactivity Disorder (ADHD)—Basic Facts *(page 4 of 4)*

Treatment of ADHD

As indicated by ADHD guidelines published by the American Academy of Pediatrics (*https://publications.aap.org/pediatrics/article/144/4/e20192528/81590/Clinical-Practice-Guideline-for-the-Diagnosis*), an effective treatment plan generally includes behavioral interventions applied at home and school, and the use of medication. The Society of Developmental and Behavioral Pediatrics (*https://sdbp.org/adhd-guideline/cag-guidelines*) recommends a life course approach to the care of children with ADHD, which means using interventions that will promote long-term skill development and independence. For this reason, it is important to focus intervention on building skills and strengthening relationships, because these are keys to long-term success and happiness. Medication frequently is an important component of a comprehensive intervention plan for children and youth with ADHD.

- Behavioral parent training
    - Especially effective for children between ages 3 and 12
    - Can be implemented effectively individually and in groups
- Classroom behavioral interventions
    - Emphasis on giving labeled praise for targeted behaviors at least four times more often than correction for unwanted behaviors
    - Daily report cards are strongly supported by research
- Child skills training
    - Training of children in organization, time management, and planning skills
    - Effective for children in grades 3–12
- Medication
    - Stimulant medication has the strongest evidence of effectiveness
    - Most children do best on a combination of psychosocial interventions and medication

Some suggestions for further reading and information for families include:

12 Principles for Raising a Child with ADHD by R. A. Barkley (Guilford Press, 2020)

Taking Charge of ADHD: The Complete, Authoritative Guide for Parents (4th Edition) by R. A. Barkley (Guilford Press, 2020)

Children and Adults with Attention-Deficit/Hyperactivity Disorder (CHADD) *https://chadd.org*

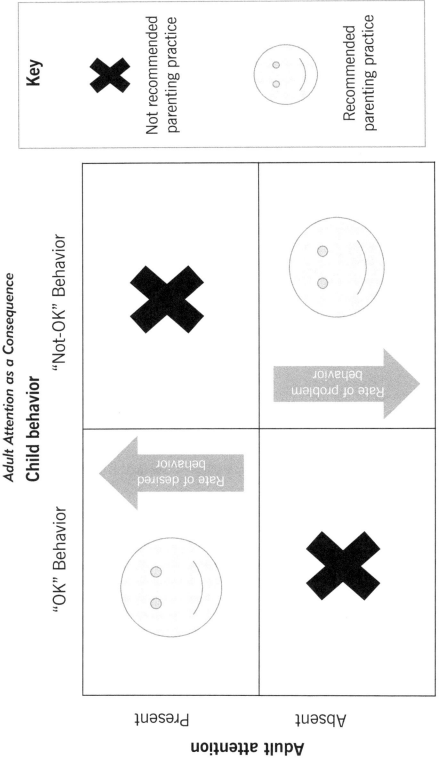

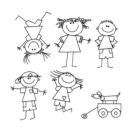

FAMILY–SCHOOL SUCCESS
SESSION 1
Catch Them Being Good

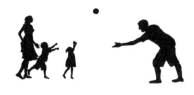

Positive reinforcement is one of the most powerful methods parents can use to improve their child's behavior. There are many forms of positive reinforcement, and we will discuss the range of positive reinforcement options in a future session.

Two of the most basic ways to provide positive reinforcement on a *frequent and immediate* basis are **positive attending** and **verbal praise.** "Catch Them Being Good" is an approach to help parents learn and practice the skills of positive attending and verbal praise.

Positive attending—observing and noticing your child's behavior and making comments describing what your child is doing that is desired and appropriate.

Examples:

Your child is playing with a building toy and while you watch, you comment, "That building is really tall."

While your child is drawing, you comment, "You are using a lot of different colors."

You smile at your child while they help a younger sibling put toys away.

Positive attending
- can be used very frequently for a wide variety of positive, desired behaviors.
- will increase the likelihood that a targeted behavior will occur more frequently.

Verbal praise—providing a compliment or positive comment to children when they perform a desired behavior or comply with a direction.

Examples:

Your child puts books back on a bookshelf, and you say, "I like when you put the books back by yourself."

While your child is playing with race cars, you say, "You are doing a great job building that race track."

Verbal praise
- is good to use when your child has complied with an instruction, followed a rule, or done something well.
- should be used often when you notice desired behavior, particularly when you are attempting to establish new behaviors.

(continued)

Catch Them Being Good *(page 2 of 2)*

Catch Them Being Good:

1. Think about behaviors your child already demonstrates that you would like to see on a more regular basis. List 3 here:

   _____
   _____
   _____

   These are your targets for positive attending (as well as appropriate play behavior or other behavior you would like to see).

2. Make positive attention comments to your child when you notice these behaviors. Take multiple opportunities throughout a day to do this. All parents/caregivers should be encouraged to use this exercise.

3. Provide verbal praise whenever your child follows an instruction, complies with a rule, or displays a behavior that is the "opposite" of an undesired behavior (e.g., shares with a sibling, cleans up toys when finished playing).

4. Set a goal of a specific number of positive attending and verbal praise statements you want to make in a day and do your best to reach your goal.

Ways I can show my child I like their behavior:

_____
_____
_____
_____
_____
_____

FAMILY–SCHOOL SUCCESS
SESSION 1

Homework—Noticing Positive/Desired Behavior

My child's positive behavior	How did I recognize the behavior?	How did my child respond?
Cleaned up his toys after playing	I said, "I like how you cleaned up your toys when you were finished!"	He smiled
Played quietly with his brother	I said, "you are doing a nice job playing very quietly."	Both boys smiled and continued playing nicely

Barriers	Strategies	How did it work?
Hard to remember to write down	Put homework sheet on kitchen table	Remembered most of the time

From *Family–School Success for Children with ADHD: A Guide for Intervention* by Thomas J. Power, Jennifer A. Mautone, and Stephen L. Soffer. Copyright © 2024 The Guilford Press. Permission to photocopy this material, or to download and print additional copies (*www.guilford.com/power2-forms*), is granted to purchasers of this book for personal use or use with students; see copyright page for details.

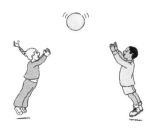
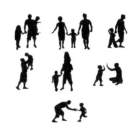

FAMILY–SCHOOL SUCCESS
SESSION 2
Child's Game

WHAT IS CHILD'S GAME?

- Child's Game is play activity between you and your child where the focus is on your child.
- **Caregiver follows, rather than leads, the child's activity** (by providing a running verbal commentary).
  - Watch closely and with interest what your child is doing. A good way to describe this is "tailgating" your child.
  - Describe enthusiastically what your child is doing. Pretend that you are a radio announcer—give a play-by-play account or a running commentary of your child's activity.
- **Caregiver attends only to "OK" behavior.** If your child does a "not OK" behavior, do not attend to it!
- Two basic types of "attends" or ways to attend to your child:
  - Describe your child's activity ("*You just put the red block on top of the green block*").
  - Praise your child for a particular "OK" behavior ("*I like how you're taking your time connecting the pieces together*").
- "Volume control" allows you to pay attention to your child in an ongoing way while increasing or decreasing the intensity of positive attention you give your child.
- When using attends:
  - Do not ask questions ("*What are you making?*").
  - Do not give any commands ("*Make the car go this way*").
  - Do not try to teach ("*Now, Kim, what are the colors in a rainbow?*").
  - Questions, commands, and teaching are ways that caregivers take control of their child's play.
  - **REMEMBER:** Your child is supposed to lead the play!

RULES FOR CHILD'S GAME

Child's Game provides an excellent opportunity for you to practice all the attending skills you've learned. It is a great way for you to strengthen the relationship you have with your child. Because children appreciate the attention they get through Child's Game, they may become more cooperative in following rules.

- Play Child's Game with your child for about 10 minutes each day, if possible. Try to make Child's Game part of your regular routine. If you cannot play Child's Game every day, try to do it 3–4 times a week.

- Allow your child to choose the activity. Toys that are well suited for Child's Game include less structured activities such as blocks and other building materials, drawing supplies, dolls, animal figures, puzzles, and toy cars and trucks. Video games and reading materials are not ideally suited for Child's Game, although they can work if the parent uses good attending skills (see above). If your child changes activities, follow along, but do not change the activity yourself.

(continued)

From *Family–School Success for Children with ADHD: A Guide for Intervention* by Thomas J. Power, Jennifer A. Mautone, and Stephen L. Soffer. Copyright © 2024 The Guilford Press. Permission to photocopy this material, or to download and print additional copies (*www.guilford.com/power2-forms*), is granted to purchasers of this book for personal use or use with students; see copyright page for details.

Child's Game *(page 2 of 2)*

- <u>Show enthusiasm when playing with your child.</u> Be careful not to take control of your child's play. You also may participate by imitating their play or following directions they give to you. Remember that your child's activity should be the center of your attention, so continue to describe their activity while working on your own.

- <u>If your child demonstrates a minor "not OK" behavior during Child's Game, ignore it.</u> However, if your child repeatedly does this, or engages in destructive or aggressive behavior, then matter-of-factly tell your child that Child's Game is over for now.

Use **PRIDE** skills with your child during Child's Game:

Praise—Tell your child specifically what you like that your child is doing.

Reflection—Restate what your child is doing in your own words.

Imitation—Join your child's play and imitate what your child is doing.

Description—Show your child how much you care by describing what your child is doing.

Enthusiasm—Make the play special by showing your enthusiasm about what your child is doing.

REMEMBER: Attending is a skill that you can use throughout the day and not just during Child's Game. Keep finding ways to pay attention to your child and give praise for "OK" behavior on a daily basis.

FAMILY–SCHOOL SUCCESS
SESSION 2

Homework—Child's Game

Date	Time (beginning–end)	Activity	Observations about self	Child response
11/5	5:15–5:30pm	Action figures	Focused on imitating; asked a few questions	Smiled, asked to play longer

Barriers	Strategies	How did it work?
Difficult finding time for Child's Game	Set a reminder on my phone	Improved consistency

FAMILY–SCHOOL SUCCESS
SESSION 3
The A-B-C Model of Behavior

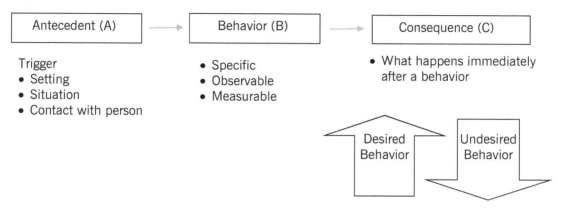

Trigger
- Setting
- Situation
- Contact with person

- Specific
- Observable
- Measurable

- What happens immediately after a behavior

- **Antecedent:** Occurs just **prior to** the behavior and makes a behavior either more or less likely to occur.

- **Consequence:** Occurs immediately **after** the behavior and causes a behavior to be more or less likely to be repeated.

- **Examples:**
  - Antecedent (A): Parent requests that children turn off the television and get ready for bed.
  - Behavior (B): Child ignores parent and continues to watch the television while siblings do as they are told.
  - Consequence (C): Parent repeatedly tells child to go to bed until the child finally listens. The unintended consequence of this is that the child gets to stay up later and gets a lot of parental attention.

The purpose of behavior therapy is to change a targeted behavior by strategically changing the antecedents and consequences of the behavior.

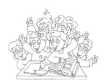

FAMILY–SCHOOL SUCCESS
SESSION 3
Effective Instructions

1. **Don't compete with the TV.** Instructions that you give should be issued with as few distractions as possible. Make sure that your child is not distracted by the television, computer, video games, or anything else when you issue a request.

2. **Maintain eye contact.** You are much more likely to have your child's attention if you make and keep eye contact.

3. **Keep instructions brief.** Given that children with ADHD typically have problems following directions, particularly those involving more than one step, it is important to issue instructions in simple statements. Limit these to one specific behavior at a time. *Example:* "Please put your books on the desk." *Not:* "Put your books on the desk, take out the worksheet, and do the first 10 problems."

4. **Use a neutral tone of voice.** Many children with ADHD are highly reactive to the emotional tone of instructions given by others. Consequently, these children often respond in an oppositional or hostile manner to the instruction, ignoring or not noticing the actual content of the message.

5. **Make it a statement!** In other words, an instruction should not be given as either a question or favor.
   Question: "Do you want to start homework now?"
   Favor: "Would you do me a favor and get out your homework book?"
   Statement: "Please begin your assignment now."

6. **Be reasonable.** Make your instructions reasonable and achievable. Don't set your child up to fail. Remember the saying "Choose your battles carefully."

7. **Mean what you say—Say only what you mean.** Show your child you mean what you say by issuing instructions firmly, and by being *prepared to follow up* on promised consequences. Remember, actions speak louder than words, despite how loudly our words can be stated. Be patient with your child's responses as you begin to use this technique. At first children are likely to test you by displaying more noncompliant behaviors. The key reasons for the increase in undesirable behaviors are:
   a) Your child will not believe you are serious until you consistently demonstrate follow-through.
   b) Your child will not initially like your reassertion of authority.

8. **Please tell me what I just said.** Tell your child to repeat each simple instruction. This may feel awkward to you at first. However, by telling your child to repeat what you have requested, you get the benefits of:
   a) Making sure you were heard.
   b) Getting feedback as to *how* your instructions are heard. For instance, you may not realize that you are giving multiple-step, complicated directions until your child attempts to repeat what you have said.

   Remember to praise your child when simple instructions are correctly repeated back to you. Also praise partial correctness (e.g., "Terrific! I did say that it is time to begin, but I said it was time to begin homework, not dinner."). If your child does not repeat your instruction at all correctly, state it again in a calm voice, and again ask them to state it back to you.

9. **Have positive consequences prepared ahead of time.** State these clearly when you issue the instruction. *Example:* "Daryl, if you finish these five math problems, you can pick a reward from this list."

10. **I am only going to say this once.** Make clear to your child how many times you are willing to repeat an instruction before you will enforce negative consequences. Our recommendation is to issue the direction, give your child 15 seconds to comply, issue a warning if necessary, and then within 5 additional seconds provide a consequence if your child does not comply.

Adapted from Power, Karustis, and Habboushe (2001). Copyright © 2001 The Guilford Press. Reprinted by permission in *Family–School Success for Children with ADHD: A Guide for Intervention* by Thomas J. Power, Jennifer A. Mautone, and Stephen L. Soffer (The Guilford Press, 2024). Permission to photocopy this material, or to download and print additional copies (*www.guilford.com/power2-forms*), is granted to purchasers of this book for personal use or use with students; see copyright page for details.

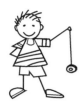
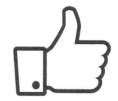

FAMILY–SCHOOL SUCCESS
SESSION 3
Understanding and Changing the Consequences of Behavior

A *consequence* is anything that <u>happens *after* a behavior occurs and has an effect on that behavior happening again</u>. Consequences may include rewards (reinforcement), punishment, or ignoring. When associated with consequences, the terms *positive* and *negative* indicate introducing something into a situation (positive) or removing something from a situation (negative).

Reinforcement

Purpose: ***increase*** the chance that a behavior will happen more often in the future.

Types of reinforcement:

Positive reinforcement: Something desired is introduced or given to the child in response to a desired behavior.

Examples:
1. Saying, "I like how you cleaned up all of your toys!" (Cleaning up toys results in verbal praise.)
2. Allowing your child extra time to watch TV after child completes homework in a reasonable period of time. (Completing homework on time earns a special privilege.)

Negative reinforcement: Something undesired is removed/avoided in response to a behavior.

Examples:
1. When you are checking out of the grocery store, your child keeps whining to get a candy bar. You give in and get your child the candy and your child stops whining. (By giving in to your child and getting the candy bar, you obtain negative reinforcement by removing or ending the whining. It should be noted that giving the candy bar positively reinforces your child for whining, which makes it more likely your child will whine in this situation in the future.)
2. You get into an argument with your child during homework when the child plays with the family pet. (By getting in an argument during homework, the child obtains the negative reinforcement of temporarily avoiding homework.)

Punishment

Purpose: ***decrease*** the chance that a behavior will happen in the future.

Types of punishment:

Positive punishment: Something negative (unpleasant, undesired) is introduced to the situation in response to a behavior.

Examples:
1. Telling your child to do an extra chore because your child hit a younger sibling.
2. Giving verbal correction when your child keeps staring out the window during homework.

(continued)

From *Family–School Success for Children with ADHD: A Guide for Intervention* by Thomas J. Power, Jennifer A. Mautone, and Stephen L. Soffer. Copyright © 2024 The Guilford Press. Permission to photocopy this material, or to download and print additional copies (*www.guilford.com/power2-forms*), is granted to purchasers of this book for personal use or use with students; see copyright page for details.

Understanding and Changing the Consequences of Behavior *(page 2 of 2)*

Negative punishment: Something positive (desired) is taken away/removed in response to a behavior.

Examples:
1. Taking away video game privileges for a half hour when your child does not start homework on time.
2. Removing access to attention from family members and privileges (time out) when your child says something hurtful to a sibling.

Ignoring (extinction)

Purpose: **decrease** the chance that a behavior will happen more often in the future.

Ignoring: A strategic decision not to pay attention to your child in response to the child's behavior.

Examples:
1. Your child nags you in order to get a cookie and you strategically respond by not paying any attention to the child.
2. Your child has a temper tantrum when being ignored, and you strategically decide to keep ignoring the child (while checking to make sure the child is safe).

FAMILY–SCHOOL SUCCESS
SESSION 3

Using Positive Reinforcement

Positive reinforcement refers to providing a consequence that makes a behavior more likely to happen again. Positive reinforcement is a very powerful tool for changing behavior and is generally preferable to punishment.

Parents often express their opinion that "my child misbehaves in order to get attention." Statements such as this reveal a common understanding that attention is a powerful reinforcer of behavior. There are many examples of how positive reinforcement plays a role in daily life. For instance, if you did not receive a paycheck for going to work and doing your job (positive reinforcement), you would probably stop going to that job. Furthermore, if your boss is someone who lets you know when you are doing a good job, you are more likely to want to work harder for that person.

A key to using positive reinforcement as a strategy for changing behavior is to selectively reinforce specific desirable behaviors, and to consistently withhold reinforcement for undesirable behaviors. For example, a reward may be given for beginning homework on time, with no reward earned for beginning homework late. Using positive reinforcement makes sense and most parents are aware of its applicability in many areas of life. However, there are often a number of challenges to consistently providing positive reinforcement with children who have ADHD.

1. **ADHD.** Children with ADHD often display more disruptive and unproductive behaviors than cooperative and responsible behaviors. Parents of children with ADHD may feel that it is difficult to find examples of cooperative behaviors to reinforce.

2. **Let sleeping dogs lie.** Many parents do not praise their child out of concern that if they do so, disruptive behaviors will soon resurface. *This concern often has a basis in fact*. The problem, however, is that when the "sleeping dog" approach is used, parents do not reinforce cooperative behavior, and may end up inadvertently reinforcing undesirable actions.

3. **I object!** Sometimes parents do not feel particularly comfortable giving rewards for their children's appropriate behaviors. These objections take several forms:
    a) *"I should not have to reward my child for things they should already be doing."* We agree: Your child *should* already be acting appropriately. However, they are *not* behaving in a way that works well in your home. *Reality check: Start with where your child is, not with where you think your child should be.*
    b) *"I'll go broke!"* As you will see, reinforcers that do not involve money are actually preferable to ones for which you must pay. The bottom line is that you are in control of the structure of this system and should feel comfortable with it.
    c) *"My child will expect to get something every time they behave well."* <u>First things first:</u> The immediate goal is to improve your child's behavior and performance. Over time you may find that you can gradually reduce the frequency of rewards and change the kinds of reinforcers you provide. For now, however, provide reinforcers very, very frequently.

(continued)

Adapted from Power, Karustis, and Habboushe (2001). Copyright © 2001 The Guilford Press. Reprinted by permission in *Family–School Success for Children with ADHD: A Guide for Intervention* by Thomas J. Power, Jennifer A. Mautone, and Stephen L. Soffer (The Guilford Press, 2024). Permission to photocopy this material, or to download and print additional copies (*www.guilford.com/power2-forms*), is granted to purchasers of this book for personal use or use with students; see copyright page for details.

Using Positive Reinforcement *(page 2 of 4)*

d) *"There's nothing my child wants."* or *"Something that's rewarding one week is ineffective the next week."* These objections highlight the need to use variety (and mystery), particularly in dealing with a child with ADHD, when providing reinforcement. For some children it will be difficult to identify effective reinforcers. Be creative, and be sure to ask your child about what they may like to earn. Ask other parents as well for reinforcer ideas.

e) *"This all takes too much time."* As with all changes in parenting routines, establishing a positive reinforcement system takes some time. As it becomes routine, little additional time will be required.

Types of positive reinforcers. There are four main categories of positive reinforcers. As you review these categories, you may note that your child responds well to different types of reinforcers in different situations.

1) *Sense of Personal Pride:* This refers to the intrinsic feelings of accomplishment an individual gets for a job well done. Although many parents believe that their child should be motivated mainly by personal pride, in many situations this type of reinforcement is not sufficient, particularly for a child with ADHD.

2) *Attention:* This pertains to involving oneself with another person in response to a particular set of behaviors. Specifically regarding a parent and child, attention can take the form of any sort of engagement with your child, in both verbal and nonverbal ways. Remember that attention can be either positive or negative. The focus here is on using positive attention. We recommend that parents use a variety of verbal and nonverbal attention reinforcers, such as:

Verbal praise and *nonverbal encouragement*
"Nice job"
"I like it when you work so hard"
"Keep up the good work"
Thumbs-up signs
Winks
Hugs
Smiles
High-fives

3) *Privileges:* Special activities that must be earned. Some examples:

Taking a trip to the park	Helping make dessert
Having a late bedtime	30 minutes of TV time
30 minutes of video game	Playing a special game
Going to the movies	Spending night with friends
Having a party	Eating out
Planting a garden	Being excused from a chore

4) *Concrete rewards:* Prizes, stickers, and tokens. Some examples:

Money	New clothes
Toys	Special snack
Mobile device apps	Select own gift
Tokens/points toward rewards	

Personal pride, attention and verbal praise, and privileges are preferable to relying on the use of concrete rewards. However, it is important to recognize that concrete rewards can be very effective, and in some cases necessary, in changing and shaping behaviors.

(continued)

Using Positive Reinforcement *(page 3 of 4)*

Reward Menu. Positive reinforcement systems tend to be more effective when children know ahead of time that they will have a <u>Reward Menu</u> from which to choose. Select a good time to sit down and tell your child, "We are going to start a program in which you can earn things. Let's start a list." If your child names an expensive item or time-consuming activity, you can direct the child to cut a picture of the item out of a magazine, or to draw a picture of the activity. The picture can then be cut into smaller pieces. Each time the child earns a reinforcer, a piece of the picture can be pasted onto a piece of paper on the refrigerator. When the picture is completed the reinforcer is earned! Also, we recommend that reinforcers be divided into:

a) Reinforcers that can be earned on a daily basis (frequent reinforcers)
b) Reinforcers that can be earned on a weekly basis (can also be used for bonuses)
c) "Bigger ticket" items that can be earned from tokens or points

Variety. Reward systems tend to become stale; therefore, it is important to vary the list frequently. An element of mystery often increases a child's motivation to increase desirable behaviors. For instance, the name of a reward can be written on a piece of paper and placed in an envelope, with the envelope labeled "Mystery Motivator." Alternately, there can be a "grab bag" of small prizes, such as those that can be purchased at a dollar store. Some parents have also found the use of a *Wheel of Fortune*–type spinner or Velcro dartboard to be helpful ways of keeping mystery and variety in the reward system, with the child receiving the reinforcer that corresponds to the number that is obtained on the spinner or board.

Bonus time! Your child should know that bonuses are always available for exceptionally good behavior. Many parents like to give a bonus for good *attitude*, such as cooperating and beginning work without being asked.

Tokens and points. Giving concrete rewards or privileges to a child each time they are productive is usually not practical. Tokens and points, on the other hand, tend to be more practical in helping parents stick to the basic principles discussed below. Some parents keep tokens in their pocket at all times, so that positive behaviors can be immediately reinforced. A handout in Session 5 will be provided that provides guidelines for using a token or point system.

Fundamental principles. Many parents have previously tried some form of positive reinforcement system. However, some of the basic principles may have been omitted. We refer to the basic system as *CISS-4:*

> **C**onsistency: Reward consistently for desirable behaviors.
>
> **I**mmediacy: As much as possible, give rewards immediately.
>
> **S**pecificity: Be very clear about what you expect.
>
> **S**aliency: Use reinforcers that are meaningful to your child.
>
> **4**-to-1 positive-to-negative ratio for responses.

Consistency. Easier said than done, we know, but reward systems usually do not work well when they are used inconsistently. With consistency both you and your child will know exactly which behaviors will be responded to and in what manner. You are also likely to find that arguments and other conflicts will be reduced.

Immediacy. Immediate positive responses to productive behaviors can make a large difference. Don't delay! For tasks that are lengthy, such as homework, provide reinforcers as soon as you notice examples of productive and attentive behaviors.

(continued)

Using Positive Reinforcement *(page 4 of 4)*

Specificity. Being very specific about what you expect and what you are reinforcing is critical. Rewarding a child for "being good" can be very confusing and does not inform the child specifically what the child has done to be reinforced. Consequently, reinforcement delivered in a nonspecific manner may not be that useful in increasing the likelihood that a child's behavior will improve. Thus instead of saying "you earned a reward coupon for being good," you may wish to say "you earned a reward coupon for following my directions without any reminders."

Saliency. Making sure that rewards are *meaningful* to your child seems like an obvious point. Families cannot afford to get too comfortable with reward systems, however, because what is meaningful to your child this month may not be very attractive next month. Remember that as your child becomes familiar with the system, your child's preferences for rewards will change.

4-to-1 Positive-to-Negative Ratio. We have already discussed how important and challenging it can be to get into the habit of giving positive reinforcement. There is a place for using punishment, as you will see in future sessions. However, even when punishments are introduced, it is vital that the frequency of positive reinforcers far outweigh that of punishments. Keeping a 4-to-1 ratio will not only make you feel more positive about managing your child's behavior, but research has shown such a ratio to be very effective. And in turn you will be more likely to be seen by your child as someone who it is good to work for, a "good boss."

Importance of practice. At this point it is important that you use positive reinforcement extremely frequently. Pay close attention to what your child is doing, and make it a point to notice the productive and cooperative behaviors. In some families this may entail giving praise or a token for complying with such commonplace parental requests as passing the salt at the dinner table. The key point here is to make a radical shift in the ratio of positive to negative feedback you are giving to your child, and to get into more positive parenting habits.

We've tried this before: It works for a week and then stops working. If you are thinking this right now, we encourage you to reread this handout and closely examine where in the CISS-4 system your previous approach may have been somewhat weak. As with the other strategies taught in this program, if you experience problems, please contact us.

Be patient! Many parents report large increases in compliance almost as soon as a positive reinforcement system is begun. However, it may take a week or more of consistently using the system before you begin to notice results. With an emphasis on "catching them being good," we are confident that over time you will begin to experience changes in behavior and an improvement in the relationship with your child.

FAMILY–SCHOOL SUCCESS
SESSION 3

Homework—A-B-C Worksheet

Antecedents	Behavior	Consequences	Outcome
What happened immediately before?	What did your child do?	What did you do?	What was your child's response to the consequence?
Younger sibling took his toy	Cried, had a tantrum	Took the toy from the sibling, gave it to child	Stopped crying, played with the toy
I said, "it's time to clean up your toys."	Cleaned up toys	I said, "I like how you follow directions the first time."	Smiled and kept cleaning up

Barriers	Strategies	How did it work?
Hard to remember to write down	Put homework sheet on kitchen table	Remembered most of the time

From *Family–School Success for Children with ADHD: A Guide for Intervention* by Thomas J. Power, Jennifer A. Mautone, and Stephen L. Soffer. Copyright © 2024 The Guilford Press. Permission to photocopy this material, or to download and print additional copies (*www.guilford.com/power2-forms*), is granted to purchasers of this book for personal use or use with students; see copyright page for details.

FAMILY–SCHOOL SUCCESS
SESSION 3
Homework—Reward Menu

Please make a list of possible rewards for your child. Remember that these rewards do not have to cost money!!

1. _____

2. _____

3. _____

4. _____

5. _____

6. _____

7. _____

8. _____

9. _____

10. _____

From *Family–School Success for Children with ADHD: A Guide for Intervention* by Thomas J. Power, Jennifer A. Mautone, and Stephen L. Soffer. Copyright © 2024 The Guilford Press. Permission to photocopy this material, or to download and print additional copies (*www.guilford.com/power2-forms*), is granted to purchasers of this book for personal use or use with students; see copyright page for details.

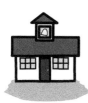
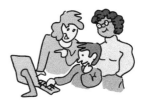

FAMILY–SCHOOL SUCCESS

SESSION 4

Tips for Building Partnerships with Teachers

- Let the teacher know that **you appreciate what the teacher is doing for your child.** It is helpful if you can acknowledge that your child presents some challenges in the classroom. Consider sending a brief note to school to let the teacher know you appreciate what they are doing for your child.

- Listen to the teacher and **identify the concerns the teacher has with your child.** Let the teacher know that you would like to assist in addressing the concerns, and select one problem to address first.

- **Analyze the problem with the teacher.** Discuss with the teacher events that may cause the problem to occur, as well as ways in which your child might be obtaining reinforcement (even if it is unintentional) for the problem behavior. Then work with the teacher to develop a plan to work on the problem. Identify tasks the teacher will implement, as well as those that you will work on.

- Develop a **plan for monitoring your child's performance** to determine whether your child is making progress. Brief teacher or parent checklists can be helpful and easy to use. You can also track progress using grades, worksheets, and homework assignments.

- **Make sure you follow through on tasks that you have agreed to accomplish.**

- Meet with the teacher periodically to **review progress** and modify the plan (if needed).

- Remember that the teacher is ultimately in charge of the school setting, and you are in charge of home. Unless the teacher asks for your advice, **telling the teacher what to do is not effective.**

- Although there may be several things the teacher is doing that you do not like, **refrain from criticizing the teacher.**

- If you find yourself getting frustrated with the teacher, refrain from being critical. **Review earlier steps and continue to provide support** and positive reinforcement to the teacher.

- When all else fails, **invite a consultant to join you** in meeting with the teacher. Make sure the teacher knows about the consultant and agrees to meet with a consultant. Consultants may be school psychologists, guidance counselors, or other teachers who are effective in working with parents and teachers.

From *Family–School Success for Children with ADHD: A Guide for Intervention* by Thomas J. Power, Jennifer A. Mautone, and Stephen L. Soffer. Copyright © 2024 The Guilford Press. Permission to photocopy this material, or to download and print additional copies (*www.guilford.com/power2-forms*), is granted to purchasers of this book for personal use or use with students; see copyright page for details.

FAMILY–SCHOOL SUCCESS
SESSION 4
Developing a Daily Report Card

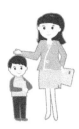

Remember the purpose of daily report cards.

1. Improve home–school communication
2. Provide the child specific, frequent feedback
3. Increase the occurrence of targeted behaviors

Draft a daily report card. Here are the steps:

1. Identify target behaviors
   - Start small (2–3 behaviors)
   - Be positive (indicate specifically what the child is to do)
   - Include target behaviors focused on academic and behavioral goals
   - Develop in collaboration with your child and with the teacher, if possible
2. Identify rating scale.
   - Ratings can be numeric. Here is an example:
     0 = try harder (met goal less than 25% of the time)
     1 = OK job (met goal 25–50% of the time)
     2 = good job (met goal 51–75% of the time)
     3 = great job! (met goal 76–100% of the time)
   - Feedback should be frequent, if possible (e.g., at the end of the morning and afternoon; after each academic period)
3. Include a place for:
   - Date
   - Parent signature
   - Teacher initials/signature
   - Parent/teacher comments
   - Total # of points earned per day
4. If you can set up a home–school meeting, work with the teacher to decide:
   - Target behaviors
   - Rating scale
   - Goal (number of points) to obtain a reward
   - Person responsible for completing the daily report card
   - Role of the child in obtaining ratings
   - How the teacher will provide feedback to the child
   - What reinforcer the child will earn for meeting the goal for the day
   - How the parent and teacher will respond if the child does not meet goal for the day

---

From *Family–School Success for Children with ADHD: A Guide for Intervention* by Thomas J. Power, Jennifer A. Mautone, and Stephen L. Soffer. Copyright © 2024 The Guilford Press. Permission to photocopy this material, or to download and print additional copies (*www.guilford.com/power2-forms*), is granted to purchasers of this book for personal use or use with students; see copyright page for details.

FAMILY–SCHOOL SUCCESS
SESSION 4

Sample Daily Report Card—NOT RECOMMENDED

Child's name: _____ Week of: _____

Directions: Rate the child on the behaviors listed below.

	Monday	Tuesday	Wednesday	Thursday	Friday
Pays attention	☺ ☹	☺ ☹	☺ ☹	☺ ☹	☺ ☹
Good behavior at recess	☺ ☹	☺ ☹	☺ ☹	☺ ☹	☺ ☹
No talking during class	☺ ☹	☺ ☹	☺ ☹	☺ ☹	☺ ☹
No disruptive behavior	☺ ☹	☺ ☹	☺ ☹	☺ ☹	☺ ☹
Total Points:					
Teacher Initials:					
Parent's Initials:					
Child's Initials:					

If I am good all week, I will get to pick out of the treasure chest!!!

Teacher Comments: _____
_____
_____

From *Family–School Success for Children with ADHD: A Guide for Intervention* by Thomas J. Power, Jennifer A. Mautone, and Stephen L. Soffer. Copyright © 2024 The Guilford Press. Permission to photocopy this material, or to download and print additional copies (*www.guilford.com/power2-forms*), is granted to purchasers of this book for personal use or use with students; see copyright page for details.

FAMILY–SCHOOL SUCCESS
SESSION 4

Sample Daily Report Card 1

Child's name: _____ Week of: _____

Directions: Rate the child on the behaviors listed below using the following scale:

0 = Work harder (met goal less than 25% of the time)
1 = Ok job (met goal 25–50% of the time)
2 = Good job!! (met goal 51–75% of the time)
3 = Great job!! (met goal 76–100% of the time)

Morning	Afternoon
Completed work in time allowed _____	Completed work in time allowed _____
Remained in seat _____	Remained in seat _____
Followed directions the first time _____	Followed directions the first time _____

Reward: _____

Total Points: _____   If I earn at least _____ points, I will earn my reward!

Teacher Comments: _____
_____

Parent Signature: _____
Parent Comments: _____
_____

From *Family–School Success for Children with ADHD: A Guide for Intervention* by Thomas J. Power, Jennifer A. Mautone, and Stephen L. Soffer. Copyright © 2024 The Guilford Press. Permission to photocopy this material, or to download and print additional copies (*www.guilford.com/power2-forms*), is granted to purchasers of this book for personal use or use with students; see copyright page for details.

FAMILY–SCHOOL SUCCESS
SESSION 4

Sample Daily Report Card 2

Child's name: _____ Week of: _____

Directions: Rate the child on the behaviors listed below.

0 = I followed the rules less than 25% of the time. I will work harder tomorrow.
1 = I followed the rules some of the time (25–50%). I did an OK job.
2 = I followed the rules a lot of the time (51–75%). I did a good job!
3 = I followed the rules almost all of the time (76–100%). I did a GREAT job!!

	Monday	Tuesday	Wednesday	Thursday	Friday
Morning					
Completed work in time allowed	0 1 2 3	0 1 2 3	0 1 2 3	0 1 2 3	0 1 2 3
Kept eyes on teacher during lessons	0 1 2 3	0 1 2 3	0 1 2 3	0 1 2 3	0 1 2 3
Afternoon					
Completed work in time allowed	0 1 2 3	0 1 2 3	0 1 2 3	0 1 2 3	0 1 2 3
Kept eyes on teacher during lessons	0 1 2 3	0 1 2 3	0 1 2 3	0 1 2 3	0 1 2 3
Total Points:					
Teacher Initials:					
Parent Initials:					

If I earn at least _____ points, I will earn my reward (_____) !!!

Teacher Comments: _____

From *Family–School Success for Children with ADHD: A Guide for Intervention* by Thomas J. Power, Jennifer A. Mautone, and Stephen L. Soffer. Copyright © 2024 The Guilford Press. Permission to photocopy this material, or to download and print additional copies (*www.guilford.com/power2-forms*), is granted to purchasers of this book for personal use or use with students; see copyright page for details.

FAMILY–SCHOOL SUCCESS

SESSION 5

Establishing a Token Economy

Establishing and using a token or point system can provide you and your child with a means of consistently and immediately reinforcing positive behaviors in a way that is practical. This handout summarizes the main points discussed in *Family–School Success* regarding the use of such systems. You are encouraged to refer to these guidelines from time to time as you use and revise your individualized system.

The first step is to decide whether you will use tokens or points. Older children (e.g., age 10 and older) and those with relatively mild ADHD may respond well to the use of points. On the other hand, younger children and those with relatively severe ADHD will often require the use of tokens. During the initial stages of your use of these reinforcement systems, do not penalize your child for undesirable behaviors by removing tokens or points. During this time "withdrawals" should only take place when your child wishes to obtain a concrete reinforcer or privilege.

Token System

1. **Introduce the system to your child.** Sit down with your child and discuss the system you are about to implement. Present this in a positive light, such as *"We are going to begin using a system to reward you for how hard you are working."* Indicate that specific behaviors will be rewarded when displayed. Have the following materials ready:
   - Tokens, chips, coins, or "bonus money" (see below)
   - A container in which the tokens will be placed when earned
   - Cardboard or colored paper on which to tape tokens or chips (e.g., tape 1 blue, 1 red, and 1 white poker chip on the paper, with their values written below them)

   Let your child know that you will work together with your child to identify the behaviors and tasks to do in order to get tokens. Indicate that one or more tokens will be placed in the container for each behavior that is displayed. For instance, a token can be earned for following a direction (e.g., "begin your homework" or "pick up your toys") with no more than one reminder. Emphasize that bonus tokens can be earned for exceptional behaviors, such as cooperation or rule-following without reminders or argument.

2. **Tokens and alternatives.** This handout refers to "tokens" but there are several alternatives that can be used. Alternatives to tokens include poker chips, coins, or "bonus money." Bonus money refers to slips of paper on which you and your child write a number of points and draw a picture. These slips can be created in increments of 1, 5, 10, and 20 "bonus dollars." Likewise, you may wish to assign values of 1, 5, and 10 points to white, red and blue poker chips, respectively. In any case, a sample of the token or alternative that is selected should be posted in a clear location.

3. **Prepare the container.** You and your child should then decorate a token container with colorful pictures or drawings. The container and tokens will be brought out during a specific time of day and will otherwise remain in a place where the parent has primary control of the tokens and container.

4. **Reward menu.** A reward menu should now be created for use with this system. The first step in creating a menu is to brainstorm reinforcer ideas. Some children will volunteer primarily expensive

(continued)

Adapted from Power, Karustis, and Habboushe (2001). Copyright © 2001 The Guilford Press. Reprinted by permission in *Family–School Success for Children with ADHD: A Guide for Intervention* by Thomas J. Power, Jennifer A. Mautone, and Stephen L. Soffer (The Guilford Press, 2024). Permission to photocopy this material, or to download and print additional copies (*www.guilford.com/power2-forms*), is granted to purchasers of this book for personal use or use with students; see copyright page for details.

Establishing a Token Economy *(page 2 of 3)*

items, which are inappropriate for daily use as reinforcers. Do not criticize your child's ideas, but if they suggest primarily expensive items, write them on the reward menu in a category labeled "longer term rewards." Then provide examples of reinforcers that can be earned on a short-term basis, such as a special dessert, 30 minutes of television or video game time, and exemption from doing a chore for the night. After the ideas have been generated, create a more formal-looking reward menu. You are encouraged to make the reward menu appear as attractive as possible. Many parents choose to create a reward menu that resembles a restaurant menu. Particularly at the outset, do not make the price of rewards overly expensive, or else your child may become discouraged and lose interest in the system. Here is a selection from a sample reward menu:

Reward	*Price*
1 hour of television	5 chips
Trip to movies	25 chips
Weekend sleepover	50 chips

5. **Identifying target behaviors.** Engage your child in a brainstorming discussion of behaviors that can earn tokens. Target behaviors can include following rules or procedures (e.g., arriving to the dinner table on time; brushing teeth for 2 minutes; starting homework at the designated time) or performing household chores (e.g., emptying the kitchen trash after dinner; putting soiled clothes in hamper before bedtime). At the outset, we suggest that you select only 3–4 target behaviors to prevent the system from becoming overly complicated. In addition, we suggest that the behaviors included in the system include at least one that is relatively easy for the child to perform, so the child will experience early success. In assigning number of tokens earned for each behavior, keep in mind that behaviors that are more difficult for your child to perform should earn more tokens. Note that it is possible to earn partial credit. For example, if the child can earn 5 chips for brushing teeth for 2 minutes, you could give your child 2 chips for brushing teeth for 1 minute. Here is an example:

Target behaviors	*Number of chips earned*
Arriving at dinner table on time	1 chip
Taking out trash after dinner	3 chips
Putting clothes in hamper before bedtime	3 chips
Brushing teeth for 2 minutes	5 chips

6. **Optional progress tools.** It may be difficult for you and your child to keep track of how many tokens have been earned, particularly if the child is seeking to earn a "big ticket" item or privilege requiring many tokens. In such cases you may wish to draw a "thermometer," which will be gradually filled in as tokens are earned. Write the name of the desired reinforcer at the top of the thermometer; when it is completely filled, the reinforcer is earned! Alternately, a picture or drawing of a desired reinforcer can be cut up into smaller "puzzle" pieces. As each piece is earned (e.g., 5 points per piece), the pieces of the puzzle are posted together until it is completed. Once completed, the reinforcer is earned.

7. **Variety: The spice of positive reinforcement.** Be sure to include variety in the way you *deliver* reinforcers.
    - *Delivery of reinforcers.* Short-term reinforcers, or items that can be issued very frequently, may be delivered by way of a *Wheel of Fortune*–type spinner, Velcro dartboard, grab bag, or "mystery motivator." Regarding the use of a spinner or dartboard, once having earned (for

(continued)

Establishing a Token Economy *(page 3 of 3)*

example) 10 points, your child may spin the wheel or toss a Velcro ball. The reinforcer that is earned will be the one upon which the wheel-pointer or ball lands. A grab bag can be filled with dollar-store items, or with slips of paper on which you have written special activities or privileges. When using a mystery motivator, an item (or slip of paper with the item or privilege written on it) is placed in an envelope. The outside of the envelope may have a question mark written on it. The envelope should be prominently placed for the child to see. Introducing an element of surprise tends to increase children's interest in positive reinforcement systems.
- *Variety of reinforcers*. It is important that the reward menu be periodically revised to ensure that only effective reinforcers are on the list. You are aware that your child's interests change over time. Thus, an item or privilege that may be a powerful reinforcer when you initially use your system may lose its effectiveness over time in promoting productive behaviors. Be sure to review the reward menu with your child on a monthly basis to add and delete items as indicated.

8. **"Dad, please give me the reward now! I promise I'll follow the rules!"** Some children will attempt to bargain with parents, saying that they will behave appropriately in the future if they can get a reinforcer immediately. To encourage your child to be more responsible, it is important that reinforcers only be delivered after the target behaviors have been displayed.

9. **How about when a reinforcer has not been earned?** If a reinforcer is not earned, do not criticize your child. Merely express hope that your child will earn the reinforcer in the future.

10. **Tip the scales toward success!** Your positive reinforcement system should be devised so that your child earns multiple tokens around 80% of the time (on average 5–6 days per week). This is important because overly stringent standards may very well discourage your child and lead to conflict and frustration. On the other hand, if your child earns many reinforcers nearly 100% of the time, there is little incentive for behavior changes.

Point System

Most of the guidelines pertaining to token systems are also appropriate when using a point system. There are a few special considerations, however.

1. **The "bank book."** Parents should create a "bank book" when planning a point system for the home. There should be columns for date, "deposit" of points, "withdrawal," and balance. You may wish to label the front of this simply as the "Home Bank Book," or use a label suggested by your child.

2. **Open for business!** A point-system bank book should be kept in your possession. To jump start the system you may wish to place 100 points (for example) in the account as a reward to your child for cooperation during the initial discussion of the point system. During periods when your child has the opportunity to earn points, display the bank book and provide a reminder about the current balance.

3. **Deposits and withdrawals.** Using a tool such as the *Home Rewards Worksheet* can help you keep track of points earned each day. When it is time to enter earned points in the bank book, you should provide supervision while your child enters points earned in the "deposit" column of the bank book. Provide similar supervision when points are withdrawn for use in purchasing reinforcers from the reward menu.

Other Considerations

If your child has siblings, you may want to create a token or point system for them as well. In such cases you are encouraged to devise a token or point system that is appropriate to the sibling's needs and developmental level.

FAMILY–SCHOOL SUCCESS

SESSION 5

Homework—Target Behaviors

- Please make a list of possible target behaviors for your child.
  - These behaviors should be <u>stated positively.</u>
    For example, "Follow directions the first time."
  - Include target behaviors that are relatively easy and difficult for your child.
- Indicate how difficult the behavior is for your child to complete.
- <u>CIRCLE</u> the 2–3 BEHAVIORS you would like to focus on for the next week.

	Target behavior	Difficulty for child
1.		
2.		
3.		
4.		
5.		
6.		
7.		
8.		
9.		
10.		

Barriers	Strategies	How did it work?
Hard to remember to write down	*Put homework sheet on kitchen table*	*Remembered most of the time*

From *Family–School Success for Children with ADHD: A Guide for Intervention* by Thomas J. Power, Jennifer A. Mautone, and Stephen L. Soffer. Copyright © 2024 The Guilford Press. Permission to photocopy this material, or to download and print additional copies (*www.guilford.com/power2-forms*), is granted to purchasers of this book for personal use or use with students; see copyright page for details.

FAMILY-SCHOOL SUCCESS

SESSION 5

Homework—Home Rewards Worksheet

Week of: _____

Point value	Target behavior	Monday	Tuesday	Wednesday	Thursday	Friday	Saturday/Sunday
	Bonus points for (write in)						
	Totals						

Total points for week: _____

Adapted from Power, Karustis, and Habboushe (2001). Copyright © 2001 The Guilford Press. Reprinted by permission in *Family–School Success for Children with ADHD: A Guide for Intervention* by Thomas J. Power, Jennifer A. Mautone, and Stephen L. Soffer (The Guilford Press, 2024). Permission to photocopy this material, or to download and print additional copies (*www.guilford.com/power2-forms*), is granted to purchasers of this book for personal use or use with students; see copyright page for details.

FAMILY–SCHOOL SUCCESS
SESSION 6
Establishing the Homework Ritual

1. **Location, location, location!** Location refers to the *where* of homework. Negotiate this with your child. There should be few distractions (e.g., television, video games, toys, siblings). However, your child should be situated where you can provide the necessary supervision, such as being able to enforce time limits and provide spot checks. For instance, a bedroom may not be sufficiently accessible to parents to monitor homework performance and offer frequent praise for productive behavior.

2. **"I wanna watch TV for a while!"** Structure and routine are helpful to children, especially those with ADHD. Set up a homework routine and try to stick to it. Try to begin work at the same time each day. Consider when your child is best able to pay attention after school. Take into account meals and after-school activities such as sports or clubs. If your child is taking medication, consider when your child is benefiting from medication and schedule homework around this. In addition, try to allow your child enough playtime at the end of homework to serve as a reward for getting work done.

3. **Time limits are vital.** Establish reasonable time limits for homework and do not let homework exceed these time limits. Imposing time limits may initially be uncomfortable for parents who are anxious about their child's academic performance. However, time limits can help children work more efficiently and reduce the amount of stress during homework. You will learn to set goals that will help your child become more and more productive over time.

4. **"Gimme a break!"** This should be decided ahead of time. We recommend only a minute or two. You may want to consider a fun minute of exercise during the break or the opportunity to get a drink of water.

5. **Use a timer.** We recommend breaking homework up into parts. Set the timer for the amount of time the child is to work on each part. For some children you may have to keep the timer out of view to minimize distraction.

6. **Use a homework kit.** We recommend that you and your child put together and maintain a homework kit. This might include the following (you and your child may wish to include additional items):

Pencils	Pencil sharpener	Pens (if appropriate)
Paper	Scissors	Eraser
Calculator	Timer (see item 5 above)	Adhesive tape

    You may wish to make a game of assembling the homework kit. Praise your child for keeping the homework kit organized.

7. **"The teacher told me we don't have any homework tonight!"** How can you be sure you know what homework has been assigned to your child? This is part of the *what* of homework. Most students are expected to use some form of a Homework Assignment Sheet. If so, you should ask your child to show you the Homework Assignment Sheet when they come home from school. This should be signed by the teacher, with "No Assignment" written in and signed when appropriate.

(continued)

Adapted from Power, Karustis, and Habboushe (2001). Copyright © 2001 The Guilford Press. Reprinted by permission in *Family–School Success for Children with ADHD: A Guide for Intervention* by Thomas J. Power, Jennifer A. Mautone, and Stephen L. Soffer (The Guilford Press, 2024). Permission to photocopy this material, or to download and print additional copies (*www.guilford.com/power2-forms*), is granted to purchasers of this book for personal use or use with students; see copyright page for details.

Establishing the Homework Ritual *(page 2 of 2)*

Schools often have websites and/or parent portals that post homework assignments, which enable parents to verify what homework has been assigned. The *what* of homework also refers to bringing home the books that are needed to complete assignments. You may want to include a space on the Homework Assignment Sheet to indicate that your child has the proper materials for homework.

8. **Remember to keep your roles clear.** Your child will at times need your help understanding the homework material. This is part of your role as *homework tutor*. Keep this job distinguished from your role as *homework supervisor*. Provide assistance to your child before and after an assignment. Your primary role during homework, however, is to be a supervisor who monitors performance and who provides frequent praise for productive behavior.

9. **Here are the rules!** Post the ground rules for the homework ritual prominently. This should include each aspect discussed above, such as when homework is to begin, where it is to be completed, and when the Homework Assignment Sheet is to be shown to the parent. Make a game of devising a clear, meaningful poster of the ritual. Use poster board or construction paper.

10. **Be persistent.** Stick to the homework ritual, although you may need to make adjustments on a week-to-week basis to account for family schedules.

FAMILY–SCHOOL SUCCESS

SESSION 6

Homework—Homework A-B-C Worksheet

Antecedents	Behavior	Consequences	Outcome
How can you set your child up for homework success?	What homework behavior did you target?	How did you reinforce?	How did your child respond to the consequence?

Barriers	Strategies	How did it work?
Example: hard to remember to use A-B-C homework sheet	Example: put homework sheet on kitchen table	Example: remembered most of the time

---

Adapted from Power, Karustis, and Habboushe (2001). Copyright © 2001 The Guilford Press. Reprinted by permission in *Family–School Success for Children with ADHD: A Guide for Intervention* by Thomas J. Power, Jennifer A. Mautone, and Stephen L. Soffer (The Guilford Press, 2024). Permission to photocopy this material, or to download and print additional copies (*www.guilford.com/power2-forms*), is granted to purchasers of this book for personal use or use with students; see copyright page for details.

FAMILY-SCHOOL SUCCESS
SESSION 6
Homework—Homework Ritual Worksheet

Where?		_____ Consistent place?
		_____ Minimal distractions?
		_____ Can I easily supervise?
When?		_____ Consistent time to begin?
		_____ Time limits?
		_____ Homework broken into segments?
		_____ Scheduled short breaks?
What?		_____ Collaboration with teacher to support child with homework?
		_____ Homework assignment sheet completed and signed by teacher?
		_____ Child has materials from school?
		_____ Child has supplies (e.g., pencils, paper)?

Adapted from Power, Karustis, and Habboushe (2001). Copyright © 2001 The Guilford Press. Reprinted by permission in *Family–School Success for Children with ADHD: A Guide for Intervention* by Thomas J. Power, Jennifer A. Mautone, and Stephen L. Soffer (The Guilford Press, 2024). Permission to photocopy this material, or to download and print additional copies (*www.guilford.com/power2-forms*), is granted to purchasers of this book for personal use or use with students; see copyright page for details.

FAMILY–SCHOOL SUCCESS

SESSION 7

Managing Time and Goal Setting

Most children with ADHD waste time well when doing homework. They will resort to all kinds of actions to avoid doing work, including teasing a sibling or pet, doodling in their notebooks, and getting into arguments with their parents. It is important to develop strategies to help your child manage time and be more productive during homework.

1. **Break it up!** Homework should be divided into subunits of relatively equal length. You can divide homework by subject area and (if homework for a particular subject is lengthy) according to the amount of work required for each subject. For example, a long assignment can be divided into two or three subunits. Keep in mind your child's attention span. Be generous about how long you think each subunit should take to complete. We have found that a simple formula for subunit length is *about 3 minutes for each grade level*. For instance, a fourth grader may have subunits of 12 minutes each.

2. **Catch your child being productive.** By breaking assignments into chunks, your child will pay attention better. At the end of each subunit, provide a quick reinforcer (e.g., praise, small reward, or points toward a privilege).

3. **Supervisor and tutor.** The distinction between your roles as supervisor and tutor is important to keep in mind. Your *primary* role is to supervise your child's homework. Your role as *tutor* should only come into play in making sure, at the outset, that your child understands the directions and how to do the assignment.

4. **Let's be realistic.** Parents sometimes report that a child's rate of homework completion and accuracy is close to 100%. However, these children may be spending 2 hours or more on homework, needing an excessive amount of parent involvement. Although this pattern may temporarily reduce parent fears of a child "falling behind," the strain on the parent–child relationship and the negative student attitudes toward schoolwork are rarely worth it. We have a tool . . .

5. **Goal-Setting Tool.** We recommend using a tool that involves setting realistic goals for homework performance and sticking to realistic time limits. The next section provides a step-by-step description of how to use this tool.

USING THE GOAL-SETTING TOOL (GST)

1. **Decide ahead of time what the reward will be when goals are met.** Present this to your child as an opportunity to earn something positive. Follow the GST guidelines for distributing points after each unit of work.

2. **Break up homework into subunits.** At first, it may seem as if you are actually increasing homework time. As the GST becomes part of the daily routine, you will see that use of the GST helps children be more productive in a shorter amount of time.

3. **Set time limits.** Decide how much time your child will be permitted for each subunit. As noted, about 3 minutes for each grade level is advised. However, feel free to adjust this time limit in order to ensure success at least 80% of the time. Write this in under "Time" in Step 1 of the GST.

(continued)

Adapted from Power, Karustis, and Habboushe (2001). Copyright © 2001 The Guilford Press. Reprinted by permission in *Family–School Success for Children with ADHD: A Guide for Intervention* by Thomas J. Power, Jennifer A. Mautone, and Stephen L. Soffer (The Guilford Press, 2024). Permission to photocopy this material, or to download and print additional copies (*www.guilford.com/power2-forms*), is granted to purchasers of this book for personal use or use with students; see copyright page for details.

Managing Time and Goal Setting *(page 2 of 2)*

4. **Set completion goals.** For each subunit, ask your child how many of the problems can be completed in the time limit. This is an opportunity for you and your child to negotiate. Based on your experience, you may know that your child is typically able to complete 5 problems in this period. However, your child may believe 10 problems is a realistic goal. Guide your child to set goals that are realistic. If necessary, you may want to compromise and agree to a goal of 6 or 7 problems. Write that in for the "# items completed" in Step 1 of the GST.

5. **Set accuracy goals.** The next step is to negotiate the *accuracy goal*. Once again, guide your child to set goals that will ensure success at least 80% of the time. Write the accuracy goal in the "# items correct" slot in Step 1 of the GST.

6. **Make sure your child understands the directions.** It is very important to make sure your child understands what to do before beginning each subunit of work. You may want to ask the child to do the first problem with you to ensure understanding of directions.

7. **Get ready!** Set the *countdown timer* for the time designed for each subunit. Instruct your child to keep working until the beeper sounds.

8. **Provide verbal praise.** While your child is working, it is important that you provide verbal praise for on-task behaviors and productive work. Remember to provide praise for specific homework behaviors. Do not respond to requests for assistance with the work during this time. If such a request is made, tell your child to keep working and that you will give assistance when the time limit is up.

9. **Direct child to evaluate work.** At the end of the time limit, compliment your child for work that was completed. Direct your child to Step 2 of the GST. Have your child write in the appropriate slot how many items they completed. You can then determine how many items have been done correctly and fill in the blank.

10. **Evaluate completion.** In Step 3 of the GST, mark whether your child exceeded the completion goal, met the goal, or did not meet the goal.

11. **Evaluate accuracy.** In Step 4, indicate whether your child has exceeded the accuracy goal, met the goal, or did not meet the goal.

12. **Count up total points.** In Step 5, add up points earned noted in Steps 3 and 4.

13. **Provide rewards!** After homework, be sure to give the reinforcer if it has been earned. If your child is not succeeding at least 80% of the time, you may need to adjust the goals.

14. **Don't go back.** Once each subunit is over, *do not go back and work on it again, even if there are inaccuracies*. It is important to get through homework without spending too much time. Write a note to the teacher indicating that your child worked independently and was not able to get all the work done correctly.

FAMILY–SCHOOL SUCCESS
SESSION 7
Goal-Setting Tool

Date: _____

Step 1. What is my goal?

    # items completed   _____

    # items correct   _____

    Time   _____

Step 2. How did I do?

    # items completed   _____

    # items correct   _____

Step 3. Did I reach my completion goal? (Circle one)

	Points
Yes, far above goal	2
Yes, I met my goal	1
No, goal not met	0

Step 4. Did I reach my correctness goal? (Circle one)

	Points
Yes, far above goal	2
Yes, I met the goal	1
No, goal not met	0

Step 5. Total points!

_____ + _____ = _____

Completion   Correctness   Total points
(from Step 3)   (from Step 4)

_____ (Check here after giving praise for effort.)

Adapted from Power, Karustis, and Habboushe (2001). Copyright © 2001 The Guilford Press. Reprinted by permission in *Family–School Success for Children with ADHD: A Guide for Intervention* by Thomas J. Power, Jennifer A. Mautone, and Stephen L. Soffer (The Guilford Press, 2024). Permission to photocopy this material, or to download and print additional copies (*www.guilford.com/power2-forms*), is granted to purchasers of this book for personal use or use with students; see copyright page for details.

FAMILY–SCHOOL SUCCESS

SESSION 8

Using Punishment Successfully

Punishment can be an effective disciplinary strategy when used thoughtfully. The emphasis of any behavioral program should be on the frequent use of meaningful positive reinforcement and the strategic use of punishment. Here are some points to keep in mind about punishment.

1. **Why punish?** The purpose of punishment is to help children learn an appropriate set of behaviors. The purpose is not for parents to express frustration or get back at the child.

2. **Possible side effects?** Punishment can be highly effective, but it can have harmful side effects if given too often or if delivered when parents are out of control. Some of the harmful side effects include teaching children to behave aggressively when frustrated, increasing child anger and defiance, and decreasing child self-esteem.

3. **When do I punish?** Punishment is often a good strategy to use for child behaviors that are major violations of family rules and do not occur frequently. Examples of behaviors to punish may include hitting a sibling or parent, throwing objects in the house, and saying something very mean to a sibling. Ignoring or deliberately not giving attention to children is usually a better strategy to use for child behaviors that occur frequently and are less serious, such as whining, making annoying noises, and interrupting conversations.

4. **How do I punish?** There are basically two ways to punish. One way is to remove positive reinforcement after an undesirable behavior, such as withdrawing parent and sibling attention and removing privileges like screen time. Another way is to apply a consequence that the child may not like. The most common example of this is giving verbal correction to a child. Another example is assigning a chore when children break the rules.

5. **How should I correct my child?** When correcting your child, keep it brief and say what you mean clearly and firmly. State what your child should do instead of what your child should not do. For example, say "You need to get back to your work," instead of "Stop looking out the window." Remember that correction is a form of punishment. Make sure to follow the *4-to-1 rule*; the amount of positive reinforcement you give should be at least four times the amount of correction (punishment).

6. **Stay calm.** Observe your reactions when punishing your child. If you deliver punishment when you are highly emotional, there is a good chance you will say or do the wrong thing. When you deliver punishment, make sure you are in control of your emotions. Sometimes it may be necessary to use anger control strategies before punishing your child.

7. **Remove your attention during punishment.** When your child is being punished and for a brief period afterward, try not to pay attention to your child. Paying attention to your child during punishment could send mixed signals and reduce the impact of the punishment.

Adapted from Power, Karustis, and Habboushe (2001). Copyright © 2001 The Guilford Press. Reprinted by permission in *Family–School Success for Children with ADHD: A Guide for Intervention* by Thomas J. Power, Jennifer A. Mautone, and Stephen L. Soffer (The Guilford Press, 2024). Permission to photocopy this material, or to download and print additional copies (*www.guilford.com/power2-forms*), is granted to purchasers of this book for personal use or use with students; see copyright page for details.

FAMILY–SCHOOL SUCCESS
SESSION 8

Punishment Discussion Questions

1. What is the purpose of punishment?

2. What are the potential adverse effects of punishment? Why do we want to avoid using punishment too much?

3. What behaviors do you punish (vs. actively ignore)?

4. What methods do you use for punishment? What are ways to remove positive reinforcement from your child?

5. What principles should we keep in mind to make sure that punishment is effective?

6. Why is it important to be calm when we give punishment? How can we help ourselves do this?

7. How do you talk to your child while you are punishing them? How about after punishment is over?

8. Should we punish a child who is dysregulated (e.g., having a tantrum)? How do we think about this?

9. How do you punish in public?

From *Family–School Success for Children with ADHD: A Guide for Intervention* by Thomas J. Power, Jennifer A. Mautone, and Stephen L. Soffer. Copyright © 2024 The Guilford Press. Permission to photocopy this material, or to download and print additional copies (*www.guilford.com/power2-forms*), is granted to purchasers of this book for personal use or use with students; see copyright page for details.

FAMILY–SCHOOL SUCCESS
SESSION 8
Homework—Using Punishment Strategically

Involve your child in a discussion to identify two behaviors that will result in punishment. In addition, discuss with your child what the punishment will be.

Target behaviors

1. _____
   _____

2. _____
   _____

Punishment

1. _____
   _____

2. _____
   _____

Barriers	Strategies	How did it work
I found myself using punishment too frequently.	*We changed the target behavior to focus on specific actions that do not occur that frequently.*	*I am using punishment less often and positive reinforcement more often.*

Adapted from Power, Karustis, and Habboushe (2001). Copyright © 2001 The Guilford Press. Reprinted by permission in *Family–School Success for Children with ADHD: A Guide for Intervention* by Thomas J. Power, Jennifer A. Mautone, and Stephen L. Soffer (The Guilford Press, 2024). Permission to photocopy this material, or to download and print additional copies (*www.guilford.com/power2-forms*), is granted to purchasers of this book for personal use or use with students; see copyright page for details.

FAMILY–SCHOOL SUCCESS

SESSION 9

How to Address Challenging Situations

1. <u>Define the problem</u> (or "not OK" behavior)
   - What does it look like?
   - How often does it happen?

2. <u>Identify a "replacement behavior"</u> (or "OK" behavior)
   - What would you like your child to be doing instead?
   - What do you want to teach your child to do in this situation?

3. <u>Identify the "A-B-C's" of the behavior</u>
   - What are the antecedents?
     - What usually happens immediately before the not OK behavior?
     - Are there times of day, locations, or people that are more likely to "set off" this not OK behavior?
   - What are the consequences?
     - What usually happens immediately after the not OK behavior occurs?
     - Common consequences that can increase not OK behaviors include parental, peer, or sibling attention; escape from a nonpreferred task or activity (e.g., getting out of doing chores); and access to something the child wants (e.g., grabbing a toy from a sibling)

4. <u>Make environmental changes</u>
   - How can you set the stage for success?
   - What changes can you make to the environment to make the OK behavior you want to see more likely to occur?

5. <u>Identify new consequences</u>
   - Your token system is a great way to provide positive reinforcement
   - Use specific, frequent, verbal praise to reward OK behavior

6. <u>If necessary, identify a punishment</u>
   - When your child performs not OK behavior, do not provide any attention
   - Consider removing a privilege as a consequence for not OK behavior
   - Remember the 4:1 ratio. Use positive reinforcement frequently

7. <u>Use organizational strategies to be consistent in using effective techniques</u>

From *Family–School Success for Children with ADHD: A Guide for Intervention* by Thomas J. Power, Jennifer A. Mautone, and Stephen L. Soffer. Copyright © 2024 The Guilford Press. Permission to photocopy this material, or to download and print additional copies (*www.guilford.com/power2-forms*), is granted to purchasers of this book for personal use or use with students; see copyright page for details.

FAMILY–SCHOOL SUCCESS
SESSION 9
Challenging Situations Worksheet

1. What's the problem? _____
   _____
   _____

2. What's the "OK behavior" you want to see? _____
   _____
   _____

3. What are the antecedents? _____
   _____
   _____

4. What are the consequences? _____
   _____
   _____

5. How can you set the stage for success? _____
   _____
   _____

6. How can you reinforce the behavior you want to see? _____
   _____
   _____

7. Is punishment appropriate? _____ If so, what is the punishment for the "not OK" behavior? _____
   _____
   _____

Barriers	Strategies	How did it work?
Hard to remember to write down	*Put homework sheet on kitchen table*	*Remembered most of the time*

From *Family–School Success for Children with ADHD: A Guide for Intervention* by Thomas J. Power, Jennifer A. Mautone, and Stephen L. Soffer. Copyright © 2024 The Guilford Press. Permission to photocopy this material, or to download and print additional copies (*www.guilford.com/power2-forms*), is granted to purchasers of this book for personal use or use with students; see copyright page for details.

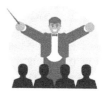

FAMILY–SCHOOL SUCCESS
SESSION 9
Maintaining Success and Anticipating Future Problems

Many images could be used to describe the challenge of successfully managing your child's behavior at home and school. At first it can seem like a juggling act, with parents struggling to use all of the different components of Family–School Success: positive attending, Child's Game, the daily report card, use of effective instructions, positive reinforcement, the A-B-C worksheets, the token economy, strategic use of punishment, and the *Tips for Building Partnerships with Teachers*. Perhaps even at this time, it is not clear how these different parts fit together. Our hope is that these components are at least starting to become part of your routine. As you integrate the parts, you should experience an improvement of your parent–child relationship, and more home and school success.

It may be most appropriate to picture all of these elements put together like a *symphony*. And like all symphony conductors, you will have to continue to pay attention to what is going on around you and make adjustments as needed. *Remember: Promoting your child's success at home and school is an ongoing process.* At times, the strategies will work nicely together and your child will respond productively and cooperatively. At other times, you may overemphasize one element (e.g., punishment) and need to make changes to accentuate another element (e.g., positive reinforcement).

Here's our "handbook" on putting it all together and looking to the future:

1. **Some progress? Any progress?** Perhaps you are fairly pleased with the progress you and your child have made over the course of this program. Or maybe you are wondering if you've actually made progress at all. It is our experience that most parents are somewhere in between feeling on top of the world about their child's behavior and feeling totally discouraged. In other words, at this point most parents report that they have made significant gains, but would still like to see improvement. Take a close look at what is going on, identify the improvements that have been made and the areas that still need work.

2. **Keep working on building a strong parent–child relationship.** Remember that a strong parent–child relationship is critical for healthy child development. Children learn how to manage their emotions and behavior through their interactions with their parents. In addition, a positive relationship with parents prepares children to have strong, positive relationships with adults and peers in school and the community. Child's Game is a helpful strategy to build a strong relationship with your child. Remember to allow your child to choose the activity and follow your child's lead during your special time together.

3. **Model learning for your child.** Family involvement in children's education contributes to school success. Families can be involved in education by working closely with school professionals and participating in school events. It is important to remember that families can also be involved in education by creating a home environment that supports learning. For example, families can make education a priority, set aside time for literacy activities, and limit television viewing. Families can also take advantage of natural learning opportunities, such as reading signs on the road, counting money while shopping, and measuring ingredients for baking.

4. **Follow the ABC's.** When a particular behavior is displayed by a child, they are usually getting something rewarding out of it, or avoiding an unpleasant situation. Antecedents (*A*'s) are what come first. Examples include how instructions are given when you need a child to complete a

(continued)

Adapted from Power, Karustis, and Habboushe (2001). Copyright © 2001 The Guilford Press. Reprinted by permission in *Family–School Success for Children with ADHD: A Guide for Intervention* by Thomas J. Power, Jennifer A. Mautone, and Stephen L. Soffer (The Guilford Press, 2024). Permission to photocopy this material, or to download and print additional copies (*www.guilford.com/power2-forms*), is granted to purchasers of this book for personal use or use with students; see copyright page for details.

Maintaining Success and Anticipating Future Problems (page 2 of 3)

task. The behaviors (*B*'s) of interest are what follow the *A*'s. Consequences (*C*'s) are responses to specific behaviors. Examples of consequences include ignoring inappropriate behaviors and praising compliance with commands. We strongly encourage an approach to behavior management that continues to look closely at the *A-B-C*'s.

5. **Give effective instructions.** Giving instructions properly is a necessary step in improving your child's behavior. Refer to the *Effective Instructions* handout, and review these tips:
   - Don't compete with the TV.
   - Maintain eye contact.
   - State instructions briefly.
   - Make it a statement.
   - Be reasonable.
   - Be prepared with consequences.
   - Mean what you say.

6. **Stay positive!** Refer to the *Using Positive Reinforcement* handout to review the basic principles of positive reinforcement. Remember how powerful your attention is, so use it strategically. Be patient, look for productive behavior, and reinforce it when you see it.

7. **Keep the token or point system going.** The *Homework—Home Rewards Worksheet* and *Establishing a Token Economy* handout can be used as tools for strengthening the positive reinforcement you provide. When used consistently, these systems should be associated with increased productivity and cooperation.

8. **Remember CISS-4.** Have we mentioned **CISS-4**? You may be tired of hearing this by now, but it is important to remember these basic principles:
   - *Consistency* is a cornerstone of behavior management. Your child must know what is acceptable and what is unacceptable. Provide positive reinforcement for desired behaviors and withhold reinforcement for undesirable behaviors. Follow these guidelines as often as you can.
   - *Immediacy* is also important. Administer consequences as soon as you can after a targeted behavior is displayed.
   - *Specificity* pertains to making it clear what will be rewarded or punished, and being precise in your responses.
   - *Saliency* refers to the meaningfulness of behavioral consequences. Reinforcers need to be valuable to the child in order for them to be effective. Remember that what is salient one week may not mean much to your child in a month or two. So be sure to keep your reward menus fresh and interesting.
   - *4-to-1* refers to maintaining a ratio of 4 positive reinforcers to 1 punishment. Do not lose sight of this ratio! Your relationship with your child will benefit, and behavioral improvements will be more consistent, with a predominantly positive approach.

9. **Use punishment sparingly and strategically.** Refer to the *Using Punishment Successfully* handout to remind yourself how to use punishment. If you find that you are slipping back into relying excessively on punishment, stop and get that positive-to-negative ratio back up to 4-to-1.

10. **Congratulate yourself!** You have probably learned some new principles to guide your child through the early years of education. In this short program you have been asked to alter many well-established patterns of parenting. If you have not reached perfection yet, don't worry. If you consistently use the principles outlined in the FSS Program, things should continue to move in a positive direction. Take time to applaud yourself and your child for the efforts you have made, the progress you have displayed, and the strategies you have mastered to meet future challenges.

(continued)

Maintaining Success and Anticipating Future Problems *(page 3 of 3)*

11. **Now what?** The following is a review of some possible problems you may encounter:
    a) **"The Blame Game."** The Blame Game is an old nemesis. It is easy for parents to forget that no one is necessarily at fault when behavioral problems appear. As discussed in this program, ADHD is related to numerous compliance problems, particularly regarding high-demand situations such as being in the classroom or completing chores. If you find yourself falling into the blame trap, take a deep breath, forgive yourself and your child, and review what you have learned here.
    b) **"The devil whispered in my ear."** When you consistently experience progress regarding your child's behavior, you may have the thought that "my child must be cured." Remember, the focus of this program has been on managing behavior, not curing it. So do not be discouraged if problems reappear. You are now in a better position to navigate the ups and downs of problem behaviors related to ADHD.
    c) **"We kept it up for a while, then it kind of faded away."** Do not let this happen to you. Perhaps the most common pitfall once a program ends is to slack off on using the strategies. Remember that you and your child did not change magically. Maintaining progress will only occur through continued hard work.
    d) **"Now they want to be rewarded for *everything*."** Remember that verbal praise and attention to positive behaviors are preferred responses. Effective behavioral approaches tend to gradually withdraw reinforcers as the desirable behaviors become more habitual for a child. One way to accomplish this is to provide concrete reinforcers less often. If you are using a token or point system, over time your child may need to earn more tokens or points in order to obtain reinforcers.
    e) **"It's hard to stay positive."** Some parents report that they have a difficult time remaining positive given their child's behavioral difficulties, even after completion of this program. We recommend that you keep a "recipe card" that outlines the CISS-4 principles and keep this well within reach. If you find yourself backsliding into giving too many punishments, keep a tally of the number of times you are giving positive reinforcement versus punishment. Increasing your self-awareness in this manner will help to change your own behavior.
    f) **"I can't seem to figure out why he does what he does."** Remember, most behaviors can be traced to getting something that is rewarding (even if it is a reprimand from a parent) or avoiding an unpleasant situation (such as beginning homework). Keep using the A-B-C worksheets to help you identify what may be sustaining a particular behavior.
    g) **"Nothing is rewarding."** We occasionally encounter children who do not respond to typical reinforcers. Parents of such children need to work harder than other parents to identify effective rewards. Of course you are encouraged to include your child in structuring and revising the reward menu. Be creative: Ask other parents, attend a local CHADD meeting (800-200-8098; *www.chadd.org*), look for internet resources, talk with your child's psychologist/therapist, and talk with your child's teacher. You are particularly encouraged to contact a mental health professional if your child's lack of response to rewards seems to be related to depressed mood.
    h) **"How often do I have to talk with my child's teacher?"** As we described throughout the program, we believe it is critically important to build effective parent–teacher relationships. Most parents find it helpful to be in regular contact with their child's teacher. Such an approach has many potential benefits, including increasing home–school consistency, receiving timely feedback regarding your child's progress, and increasing parental involvement in learning.
    i) **"Where the heck did this come from?"** Some problems will arise that you simply cannot anticipate. From time to time you will encounter new and "interesting" problems. However, the principles you have learned in this program should serve as guidelines for meeting unanticipated challenges.
12. **Now go treat yourself to a reward when the session is over! Thank you for all of your hard work during the program!**

FAMILY SCHOOL SUCCESS
SESSION 9
Formula for Success

Directions: Create an individualized plan to promote adaptive child behavior, support positive parent–child interactions, foster learning at home, and build a collaborative relationship with teachers.

1. FSS strategies that were most helpful to my family included:

   _____   _____
   _____   _____
   _____   _____

2. Tips to adapt strategies to my situation:

   _____   _____
   _____   _____

3. Organizational strategies to help me use FSS strategies consistently:

   _____   _____
   _____   _____

Formula for Success

To address behavior management

✓ At home:

_____ + _____ + _____
_____ + _____ + _____
_____ + _____ + _____

✓ At school:

_____ + _____ + _____
_____ + _____ + _____
_____ + _____ + _____

**Remember Organizational Strategies to help you use these interventions consistently!

To build a collaborative relationship with teachers

_____ + _____ + _____
_____ + _____ + _____
_____ + _____ + _____

**Remember Organizational Strategies to help you use these interventions consistently!

(continued)

Formula for Success *(page 2 of 2)*

Formula for Success Examples:

To address behavior management

At home: Keep an A-B-C worksheet on the fridge for use when needed + identify behavioral targets + continue to use token economy and positive reinforcement + regularly update rewards menu with child input + tailor token economy system to each child + "Catch them being good!" + "Catch my partner being good" (notice when partner uses FSS strategies with our children) + use an electronic calendar to remind me to provide rewards to my child.

To build a collaborative relationship with teachers

At school: Meet with new teacher early in the fall + share ideas/strategies with teacher that have helped in the past + elicit ideas from teacher + develop new home–school note + implement and modify as needed + develop a plan to ensure that the note makes it home from school daily + hang a copy of the note on the fridge as a reminder to discuss the note with my child and provide rewards contingent on goal attainment.

FAMILY–SCHOOL SUCCESS
SESSION 9
Finding a Provider for Behavior Management with ADHD

What is a "behavioral" approach to working with ADHD?

Behavioral approaches to managing ADHD are one of the two methods that are well established for treating ADHD (the other is stimulant medication). Behavioral approaches may be implemented at home and in school. Behavioral approaches identify specific problem behaviors (e.g., bringing home assignments, noncompliance) that impact a child's functioning at home and school. Once these behaviors are identified, specific strategies are developed to promote replacement behaviors. These strategies involve changing aspects of the environment (e.g., sitting closer to the teacher, reducing distractions) and modifying the consequences of behavior (e.g., rewarding positive behaviors, loss of privileges for undesirable behaviors).

How does a behavioral approach differ from other approaches?

Because behavioral approaches emphasize changing aspects of the environment or consequences for behavior, they generally require the active involvement of parents and teachers. Although a provider will likely work directly with your child, you can also expect that a significant portion of the treatment will involve working with parents and other caregivers. A therapist may only spend an hour a week with your child, but parents and teachers spend an enormous amount of time with the child. Therefore, to maximize the impact of treatment, behavioral approaches focus on helping parents and teachers develop the skills to work effectively with the child. In some sense, the therapist may serve as a coach to parents—a person to help guide them through the challenges of addressing their child's behavior.

How can I tell if a provider uses a behavioral approach?

Unfortunately, it is not always easy to tell what kind of approach a particular therapist will use and sometimes the term *behavioral* is used inconsistently to refer to a wide range of strategies. Many times, a parent only has a list of providers from their health insurance carrier and little guidance to select among them. Some characteristics are important no matter what approach a therapist uses. For instance, you should feel comfortable with the therapist and be sure that they have appropriate experience and credentials. However, here are some questions that can help you select an appropriate therapist.

- *Could you describe your general approach to working with children with ADHD?* Behavioral approaches emphasize increasing the occurrence of desirable behaviors in addition to reducing undesirable behaviors. Most effective behavioral treatment programs tend to work on increasing desirable behaviors <u>before</u> addressing undesirable behaviors. If a provider only describes strategies for addressing problem behaviors (e.g., using time out), ask them about the role of rewarding appropriate behavior.

- *Do you work primarily with the child or with the parent(s) as well?* As mentioned above, providers who work almost exclusively with the child are probably not using a behavioral approach. Behavioral intervention involves active involvement with parents and teachers to ensure they have the strategies to work effectively with children. It is important to note, however, that spending more time individually with the child may be appropriate depending on the specific needs of the child (e.g., training children in organizational skills or helping children cope with anxiety).

(continued)

From *Family–School Success for Children with ADHD: A Guide for Intervention* by Thomas J. Power, Jennifer A. Mautone, and Stephen L. Soffer. Copyright © 2024 The Guilford Press. Permission to photocopy this material, or to download and print additional copies (*www.guilford.com/power2-forms*), is granted to purchasers of this book for personal use or use with students; see copyright page for details.

Finding a Provider for Behavior Management with ADHD *(page 2 of 2)*

- *To what extent are you willing to work with my child's school?* In general, more involvement with the school is desirable. Some providers may not routinely involve the school, whereas others get involved to facilitate family–school collaboration. In some cases, the provider may be willing to visit the school to observe behavior, consult with teachers, or facilitate communication between family and school.

- *What percentage of your practice focuses on children with difficulties similar to my child's?* It is often a good idea to inquire about a therapist's level of experience. It may be helpful to ask how long the therapist has been practicing. Perhaps more important, you may also want to ask about the therapist's level of experience with the specific issues for which you are seeking help. Many mental health professionals will work with a wide range of presenting problems. It is generally desirable to find providers who spend more time working with children and families who are likely to share some of your concerns and challenges (e.g., ADHD, learning disabilities, anxiety).

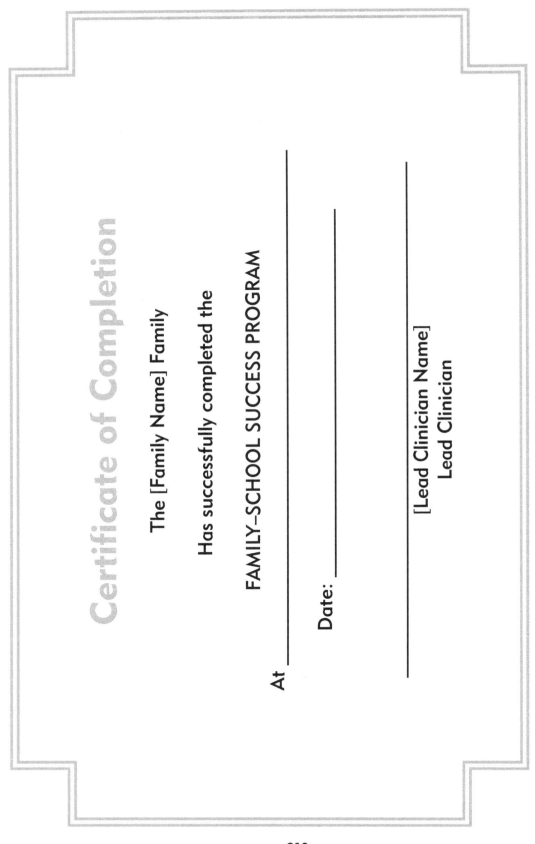

From *Family–School Success for Children with ADHD: A Guide for Intervention* by Thomas J. Power, Jennifer A. Mautone, and Stephen L. Soffer. Copyright © 2024 The Guilford Press. Permission to photocopy this material, or to download and print additional copies (*www.guilford.com/power2-forms*), is granted to purchasers of this book for personal use or use with students; see copyright page for details.

FAMILY–SCHOOL SUCCESS (FSS) PROGRAM
Template for Report of Progress

Name of Child:

Date of Birth of Child:

Informant:

Date of Report:

This report describes outcomes for the child and family in response to their recent participation in the Family–School Success program. This program is a multifamily group intervention that includes standard elements of behavioral parent training in addition to behavioral homework interventions, and a classroom behavioral intervention (daily report card). This program is usually delivered in 8–9 sessions and can be provided to families in person or by telehealth. The following sections describe your child's progress in the program assessed by several measures given preintervention, postintervention, and follow up (3 months after intervention ended). It was noted that your family attended **[insert number here]** of the **[insert number here]** sessions scheduled, which were offered **[indicate in-person or telehealth]**.

Parent Report

Domain assessed: Parent–Child Relationship

Measure administered: Parent–Child Relationship Questionnaire (PCRQ). This measure includes two scales assessing parent perceptions of their parenting practices. One scale assesses negative/ineffective parenting and the other scale assesses positive parenting. Scores can be converted to a summary score (ranging from 1 to 5). Lower scores for negative/ineffective parenting are better and indicate less negative parenting. Higher scores for positive parenting are better and indicate more positive parenting. A change in score of 0.5 of a point is considered meaningful.

Negative/Ineffective Parenting

Date completed	Mean item score
Preintervention (date)	
Postintervention (date)	
Follow-up (date)	

Positive Parenting

Date completed	Mean item score
Preintervention (date)	
Postintervention (date)	
Follow-up (date)	

Interpretation:

(continued)

From *Family–School Success for Children with ADHD: A Guide for Intervention* by Thomas J. Power, Jennifer A. Mautone, and Stephen L. Soffer. Copyright © 2024 The Guilford Press. Permission to photocopy this material, or to download and print additional copies (*www.guilford.com/power2-forms*), is granted to purchasers of this book for personal use or use with students; see copyright page for details.

Template for Report of Progress *(page 2 of 5)*

Domain assessed: Quality of the Parent–Teacher Relationship

Measure administered: Parent–Teacher Involvement Questionnaire (PTIQ). This measure is used to assess the parent–teacher relationship from the parent perspective. The measure yields a summary score (ranging from 0 to 4), with higher ratings indicating a better parent–teacher relationship. A change of 0.5 of a point is considered meaningful.

Quality of the Parent–Teacher Relationship

Date completed	Mean item score
Preintervention (date)	
Postintervention (date)	
Follow-up (date)	

Interpretation:

Domains assessed: ADHD Symptoms, Anxiety/Depression, Disruptive Behavior

Measure administered: Behavioral Health Checklist (BHCL). This parent-report measure has two sections. The first section assesses three domains: ADHD symptoms, anxiety/depression symptoms, and disruptive behaviors. The second section assesses child strengths in interpersonal relationships and self-control. Scores on these scales are converted to percentile scores. Lower scores for ADHD symptoms, anxiety/depression, and disruptive behavior indicate fewer problems. Higher scores on the child's strengths domain indicate more strengths. A change of 0.5 points is considered meaningful (lower scores reflect improvement for all scales except Child Strengths).

ADHD Symptoms

Date completed	Mean item score
Preintervention (date)	
Postintervention (date)	
Follow-up (date)	

Anxiety/Depression Symptoms

Date completed	Mean item score
Preintervention (date)	
Postintervention (date)	
Follow-up (date)	

Disruptive Behaviors

Date completed	Mean item score
Preintervention (date)	
Postintervention (date)	
Follow-up (date)	

(continued)

Template for Report of Progress (page 3 of 5)

Child Strengths

Date completed	Mean item score
Preintervention (date)	
Postintervention (date)	
Follow-up (date)	

Interpretation:

Domains assessed: Child Impairment in Academic, Interpersonal and Emotional Functioning

Measure administered: Impairment Rating Scale (IRS). This parent-report measure assesses whether a child is experiencing problems in several domains of functioning, including relationships with peers, relationships with parents, academic performance, self-esteem, and family functioning. This measure yields a summary score (ranging from 0 to 6) with lower scores indicating less overall impairment. A change of 0.5 point is considered meaningful.

Child Impairment:

Date completed	Mean item score
Preintervention (date)	
Postintervention (date)	
Follow-up (date)	

Interpretation:

Domain assessed: Homework Performance

Measure administered: Homework Performance Questionnaire—Parent Version (HPQ-P). This parent-report measure assesses understanding of homework, organization, and productivity in completing homework. This scale can be converted to a summary score (ranging from 0 to 3), with higher scores indicating better homework performance. An increase of 0.5 point is considered meaningful.

Homework Performance

Date completed	Mean item score
Preintervention (date)	
Postintervention (date)	
Follow-up (date)	

Interpretation:

(continued)

Template for Report of Progress *(page 4 of 5)*

Teacher Report

Domains assessed: Child Academic Performance

Measure administered: Academic Proficiency Scale (APS). This teacher-report measure assesses proficiency in academic subjects relative to standard expectations. Academic areas are rated on a scale from 1 to 5 (1 = well below standard expected at this time of year; 3 = at the standard; and 5 = well above the standard). This measure yields an average item score with higher scores indicating higher performance. A change in average item score of 0.5 point is considered meaningful.

Child Academic Performance:

Date completed	Mean item score
Preintervention (date)	
Postintervention (date)	
Follow-up (date)	

Interpretation:

Domains assessed: Child Impairment in Academic and Interpersonal Functioning

Measure administered: Impairment Rating Scale (IRS)—Teacher Version. This teacher-report measure assesses whether a child is experiencing problems in several domains of functioning, including relationships with peers, relationship with teacher, academic progress, self-esteem, influence on classroom functioning, and overall severity of the problem. This measure yields an average item score ranging from 0 to 6, with higher scores indicating more overall impairment. A change in average item score of 0.5 point is considered meaningful.

Child Impairment:

Date completed	Mean item score
Preintervention (date)	
Postintervention (date)	
Follow-up (date)	

Interpretation:

Domain assessed: Homework Performance

Measure administered: Homework Performance Questionnaire—Teacher Version (HPQ-T). This teacher-rated measure assesses child understanding of homework, organization, and productivity in completing homework. Each item is rated on a 7-point scale to reflect the percentage of time that each behavior occurs (0 = 0–10%; 6 = 91–100%). This measure yields an average item score rating from 0 to 6, with higher scores indicating better homework performance. A change in average item score of 0.5 point is considered meaningful.

(continued)

Template for Report of Progress (page 5 of 5)

Homework Performance

Date completed	Mean item score
Preintervention (date)	
Postintervention (date)	
Follow-up (date)	

Interpretation:

Overall Summary

Domains in which there was improvement:

Domains in which there was no change:

Domains in which there was a decline:

Recommendations

Parents/caregivers may wish to share this report with their child's primary care clinician as well as school staff.

Parents/caregivers are strongly encouraged to continue using the strategies discussed in the Family–School Success program. In particular, each family developed a formula for success, indicating the strategies that were most useful in helping their child with challenges at home and school. Parents/caregivers are strongly advised to reflect on their formula for success and implement the strategies that are most useful to them on a consistent basis.

APPENDIX B

Fidelity Checklists

Fidelity Checklist for FSS Session 1	219
Fidelity Checklist for FSS Session 2	220
Fidelity Checklist for FSS Session 3	221
Fidelity Checklist for FSS Session 4	222
Fidelity Checklist for FSS Session 5	223
Fidelity Checklist for FSS Session 6	224
Fidelity Checklist for FSS Session 7	225
Fidelity Checklist for FSS Session 8	226
Fidelity Checklist for FSS Session 9	227
Family–School Success—Process Fidelity Checklist	228

Fidelity Checklist for FSS Session 1

FSS Clinician: _____ Date: _____

Coder Name: _____

Rate each item: 0 = Not Implemented; 1 = Implemented

Introduction	Score
1. Introduced group leaders and asked parents to introduce themselves	0 1
2. Described program expectations	0 1
3. Explained the importance of maintaining confidentiality	0 1
4. Encouraged parents to inform clinicians about safety issues	0 1
5. Explained the "big ideas" of FSS	0 1

Understanding ADHD	Score
6. Discussed how ADHD has an impact on their children's performance and behavior	0 1
7. Discussed ADHD presentations, functional impairments, and comorbid conditions	0 1
8. Described evidence-based interventions for ADHD	0 1

Family Involvement in Education	Score
9. Discussed how parents can help their children do well in school	0 1
10. Discussed the importance of family–school collaboration	0 1

Positive Attending	Score
11. Discussed how parent attention influences child behavior	0 1
12. Discussed the importance of catching the child being good	0 1
13. Introduced ignoring as a strategy to reduce unwanted behaviors	0 1

Session Wrap-Up	Score
14. Prepared parents to implement homework assignments	0 1
15. Distributed handouts and homework assignments to parents	0 1

From *Family–School Success for Children with ADHD: A Guide for Intervention* by Thomas J. Power, Jennifer A. Mautone, and Stephen L. Soffer. Copyright © 2024 The Guilford Press. Permission to photocopy this material, or to download and print additional copies (*www.guilford.com/power2-forms*), is granted to purchasers of this book for personal use or use with students; see copyright page for details.

Fidelity Checklist for FSS Session 2

FSS Clinician: _____ Date: _____

Coder Name: _____

Rate each item: 0 = Not Implemented; 1 = Implemented

Homework Review	Score
1. Reviewed homework with families	0 1
2. Discussed barriers to homework completion	0 1

Caregiver Coping Strategies and Partnerships	Score
3. Discussed parents' organizational strategies to promote effective parenting	0 1
4. Discussed parents' strategies to manage their emotions when parenting	0 1
5. Discussed how to work with other caregivers to cope with the challenges of parenting	0 1

Child's Game	Score
6. Modeled Child's Game for parents	0 1
7. Discussed with parents what to do during Child's Game (PRIDE skills)	0 1
8. Discussed with parents what not to do during Child's Game	0 1
9. Provided parents an opportunity to practice Child's Game in session	0 1
10. Discussed with parents how to implement Child's Game at home with their children	0 1

Session Wrap-Up	Score
11. Prepared parents to implement homework assignment	0 1
12. Distributed handouts and homework assignment to parents	0 1

From *Family–School Success for Children with ADHD: A Guide for Intervention* by Thomas J. Power, Jennifer A. Mautone, and Stephen L. Soffer. Copyright © 2024 The Guilford Press. Permission to photocopy this material, or to download and print additional copies (*www.guilford.com/power2-forms*), is granted to purchasers of this book for personal use or use with students; see copyright page for details.

Fidelity Checklist for FSS Session 3

FSS Clinician: _____ Date: _____

Coder Name: _____

Rate each item: 0 = Not Implemented; 1 = Implemented

Homework Review	Score	
1. Reviewed homework with families	0	1
2. Discussed barriers to homework completion	0	1

ABC's of Behavior Change	Score	
3. Discussed the A-B-C model	0	1
4. Applied the A-B-C model to a specific child behavior	0	1

Antecedent and Consequence Strategies	Score	
5. Discussed ways to give effective instructions	0	1
6. Discussed the difference between positive and negative reinforcement	0	1
7. Discussed how negative reinforcement maintains maladaptive child and parent behaviors	0	1
8. Discussed the difference between positive reinforcement and bribery	0	1
9. Discussed the difference between ignoring and punishment	0	1
10. Discussed varying types of positive reinforcement	0	1

Session Wrap-Up	Score	
11. Prepared parents to implement homework assignments	0	1
12. Distributed handouts and homework assignments to parents	0	1

From *Family–School Success for Children with ADHD: A Guide for Intervention* by Thomas J. Power, Jennifer A. Mautone, and Stephen L. Soffer. Copyright © 2024 The Guilford Press. Permission to photocopy this material, or to download and print additional copies (*www.guilford.com/power2-forms*), is granted to purchasers of this book for personal use or use with students; see copyright page for details.

Fidelity Checklist for FSS Session 4

FSS Clinician: _____ Date: _____

Coder Name: _____

Rate each item: 0 = Not Implemented; 1 = Implemented

Homework Review	Score
1. Reviewed homework with families	0 1
2. Discussed barriers to homework completion	0 1

Home–School Collaboration	Score
3. Discussed the importance of the teacher–student relationship	0 1
4. Discussed how parent–teacher collaboration can influence the teacher–student relationship	0 1

Building Partnerships with Teachers	Score
5. Discussed parents' current relationships with teachers	0 1
6. Discussed strategies for strengthening family–school partnerships	0 1

Daily Report Cards	Score
7. Discussed elements of a poorly designed daily report card (DRC)	0 1
8. Discussed elements of a well-designed DRC	0 1
9. Discussed how to design a DRC for their child	0 1
10. Discussed the importance of involving the child and teacher in designing a DRC	0 1

Session Wrap-Up	Score
11. Prepared parents to implement homework assignments	0 1
12. Distributed handouts and homework assignments to parents	0 1

From *Family–School Success for Children with ADHD: A Guide for Intervention* by Thomas J. Power, Jennifer A. Mautone, and Stephen L. Soffer. Copyright © 2024 The Guilford Press. Permission to photocopy this material, or to download and print additional copies (www.guilford.com/power2-forms), is granted to purchasers of this book for personal use or use with students; see copyright page for details.

Fidelity Checklist for FSS Session 5

FSS Clinician: _____ Date: _____

Coder Name: _____

Rate each item: 0 = Not Implemented; 1 = Implemented

Homework Review	Score	
1. Reviewed homework with families	0	1
2. Discussed barriers to homework completion	0	1

Positive Reinforcement	Score	
3. Reviewed the importance of using positive reinforcement	0	1
4. Reviewed types of positive reinforcement	0	1

Token Economy	Score	
5. Discussed the value added by using a token economy system	0	1
6. Generated a menu of possible rewards that differ by frequency of delivery	0	1
7. Identified target behaviors that differ in level of difficulty for the child	0	1
8. Discussed how to assign a value to target behaviors	0	1
9. Discussed the exchange system	0	1
10. Discussed potential challenges with implementing a token system	0	1

Session Wrap-Up	Score	
11. Prepared parents to implement homework assignments	0	1
12. Distributed handouts and homework assignments to parents	0	1

From *Family–School Success for Children with ADHD: A Guide for Intervention* by Thomas J. Power, Jennifer A. Mautone, and Stephen L. Soffer. Copyright © 2024 The Guilford Press. Permission to photocopy this material, or to download and print additional copies (*www.guilford.com/power2-forms*), is granted to purchasers of this book for personal use or use with students; see copyright page for details.

Fidelity Checklist for FSS Session 6

FSS Clinician: _____ Date: _____

Coder Name: _____

Rate each item: 0 = Not Implemented; 1 = Implemented

Homework Review	Score
1. Reviewed homework with families	0 1
2. Discussed barriers to homework completion	0 1

A-B-C's of Homework Behavior	Score
3. Discussed the A-B-C's of homework performance	0 1
4. Discussed antecedent and consequence strategies to promote homework success	0 1

Establishing a Homework Ritual	Score
5. Introduced the three Ws of homework completion (where, when, what)	0 1
6. Discussed the where of homework and ideas for selecting the right place for homework	0 1
7. Discussed the when of homework and ideas for selecting the right time for homework	0 1
8. Discussed the what of homework and how to ensure the child knows what to do for homework	0 1
9. Discussed strategies for helping children organize homework materials	0 1
10. Discussed how parent–teacher communication can set the child up for homework success	0 1

Session Wrap-Up	Score
11. Prepared parents to implement homework assignments	0 1
12. Distributed handouts and homework assignments to parents	0 1

From *Family–School Success for Children with ADHD: A Guide for Intervention* by Thomas J. Power, Jennifer A. Mautone, and Stephen L. Soffer. Copyright © 2024 The Guilford Press. Permission to photocopy this material, or to download and print additional copies (*www.guilford.com/power2-forms*), is granted to purchasers of this book for personal use or use with students; see copyright page for details.

Fidelity Checklist for FSS Session 7

FSS Clinician: _____ Date: _____

Coder Name: _____

Rate each item: 0 = Not Implemented; 1 = Implemented

Homework Review	Score
1. Reviewed homework with families	0 1
2. Discussed barriers to homework completion	0 1

Importance of Time Management and Goal Setting	Score
3. Discussed the importance of placing time limits on homework completion	0 1
4. Discussed parental concerns about stopping homework at the end of established time limits	0 1
5. Discussed the importance of communicating with teachers about homework expectations and time limits	0 1

Goal-Setting Tool	Score
6. Modeled the goal-setting tool	0 1
7. Discussed parents' reactions to and questions about the goal-setting tool	0 1
8. Provided parents an opportunity to practice using the goal-setting tool	0 1
9. Discussed parents' experience in using the goal-setting tool	0 1
10. Discussed ways to adapt the goal-setting tool for use with their children	0 1

Session Wrap-Up	Score
11. Prepared parents to implement homework assignments	0 1
12. Distributed handouts and homework assignments to parents	0 1

From *Family–School Success for Children with ADHD: A Guide for Intervention* by Thomas J. Power, Jennifer A. Mautone, and Stephen L. Soffer. Copyright © 2024 The Guilford Press. Permission to photocopy this material, or to download and print additional copies (*www.guilford.com/power2-forms*), is granted to purchasers of this book for personal use or use with students; see copyright page for details.

Fidelity Checklist for FSS Session 8

FSS Clinician: _____ Date: _____

Coder Name: _____

Rate each item: 0 = Not Implemented; 1 = Implemented

Homework Review	Score
1. Reviewed homework with families	0 1
2. Discussed barriers to homework completion	0 1

Punishment Strategies	Score
3. Discussed the purpose and potential benefits of punishment	0 1
4. Discussed potential adverse effects of punishment	0 1
5. Discussed differences between punishment and ignoring	0 1
6. Discussed two main ways to punish (removing positive reinforcement and applying aversive consequences)	0 1
7. Discussed how verbal correction is a form of punishment	0 1
8. Discussed at least 3 of 5 principles in applying punishment—consistency, immediacy, specificity, saliency, and 4:1 ratio of positive to correction feedback	0 1
9. Discussed the importance of parental emotional control when delivering punishment	0 1
10. Discussed recommended parental actions during and after punishment	0 1

Session Wrap-Up	Score
11. Prepared parents to implement homework assignments	0 1
12. Distributed handouts and homework assignments to parents	0 1

From *Family–School Success for Children with ADHD: A Guide for Intervention* by Thomas J. Power, Jennifer A. Mautone, and Stephen L. Soffer. Copyright © 2024 The Guilford Press. Permission to photocopy this material, or to download and print additional copies (*www.guilford.com/power2-forms*), is granted to purchasers of this book for personal use or use with students; see copyright page for details.

Fidelity Checklist for FSS Session 9

FSS Clinician: _____ Date: _____

Coder Name: _____

Rate each item: 0 = Not Implemented; 1 = Implemented

Homework Review	Score
1. Reviewed homework with families	0 1
2. Discussed barriers to homework completion	0 1

Addressing Future Challenges	Score
3. Discussed a framework for addressing challenging situations in the future	0 1

Punishment Strategies	Score
4. Discussed how to punish children when they are dysregulated	0 1
5. Discussed strategies for punishing children in public places	0 1

Session Wrap-Up	Score
6. Identified which FSS strategies have been most helpful for each family	0 1
7. Discussed the importance of preparing a formula for success to address future problems	0 1
8. Provided parents an opportunity to prepare and discuss their formula for success	0 1
9. Discussed how to obtain follow-up support and intervention, if necessary	0 1
10. Celebrated the successes families have had	0 1

From *Family–School Success for Children with ADHD: A Guide for Intervention* by Thomas J. Power, Jennifer A. Mautone, and Stephen L. Soffer. Copyright © 2024 The Guilford Press. Permission to photocopy this material, or to download and print additional copies (*www.guilford.com/power2-forms*), is granted to purchasers of this book for personal use or use with students; see copyright page for details.

Family–School Success—Process Fidelity Checklist

FSS Clinician: _____   Coder name: _____

Session: _____   Date: _____

For each section of the session (see below), read each item and think about which description better fits the group-process variable being assessed: the description on the left side or the description on the right side. After that, decide whether the description you chose for this group process variable is "sort of true" or "really true." Thus, for each item, you'll check one of the four boxes.

| **Section # (circle one):** | 1 = "Introduction/Homework Review" part of the session |
| | 2 = "New Content" part of the session |

Really True	Sort of True				Really True	Sort of True
\multicolumn{7}{l}{**1. ENCOURAGING PARENT ACTIVE ENGAGEMENT**}					
		Facilitator's presentation was didactic (most of the talking done by the facilitator); did not try to adapt the material to individual situations	OR	Facilitator used open-ended questions, affirmations, reflections, and summaries to encourage parent engagement; adapted material to individual situations		
\multicolumn{7}{l}{**2. ELICITING AND STRENGTHENING CHANGE TALK**}					
		Facilitator focused on sustain talk or status quo (e.g., reasons parents can't do the between-session homework) without evoking and reflecting the parents' own efforts or stated reasons to change	OR	Facilitator affirmed parents' desire, ability, reasons, and need for change (e.g., completing between-session homework)		
\multicolumn{7}{l}{**3. PROVIDING EMOTIONAL VALIDATION**}					
		Facilitator was not responsive to or was critical of parents' concerns	OR	Facilitator provided social support, emotional reassurance, or validation of parents' feelings		
\multicolumn{7}{l}{**4. BUILDING CONNECTIONS AMONG PARENTS**}					
		Facilitator did not attempt to connect parents to each other	OR	Facilitator built connections among parents and built on parents' shared experiences		
\multicolumn{7}{l}{**5. MAINTAINING PARENTS' FOCUS ON FSS PRINCIPLES AND INTERVENTION COMPONENTS**}					
		Facilitator did not keep parents focused on FSS principles and components during off-topic discussions or when parents suggested something that would be contraindicated by FSS (e.g., pro-corporal punishment, negative parenting)	OR	Facilitator kept parents focused on FSS principles and components during off-topic discussions or when parents suggested something that would be contraindicated by FSS (e.g., pro-corporal punishment, negative parenting)		

Copyright © 2022 Children's Hospital of Philadelphia. Adapted and reprinted with permission of the developers (J. D. Nissley-Tsiopinis, S. Normand, J. A. Mautone, J. Fogler, and T. J. Power) in *Family–School Success for Children with ADHD: A Guide for Intervention* by Thomas J. Power, Jennifer A. Mautone, and Stephen L. Soffer (The Guilford Press, 2024). Permission to photocopy this material, or to download and print additional copies (*www.guilford.com/power2-forms*), is granted to purchasers of this book for personal use or use with students; see copyright page for details.

APPENDIX C

Outcome Measures

Parent–Child Questionnaire	231
Behavioral Health Checklist (Ages 4–7)	233
Behavioral Health Checklist (Ages 8–12)	234
Homework Performance Questionnaire (for Parents)	235
Cuestionario Sobre Desempeño en las Tareas/Asignaciones (para Padres)	237
Homework Performance Questionnaire (for Teachers)	239
Academic Proficiency Scale (APS)	242
Family–School Success Program Evaluation Scale	243
Coding Manual for Family–School Success Between-Session Homework Assignments	245
Scoring Key for Measures	248

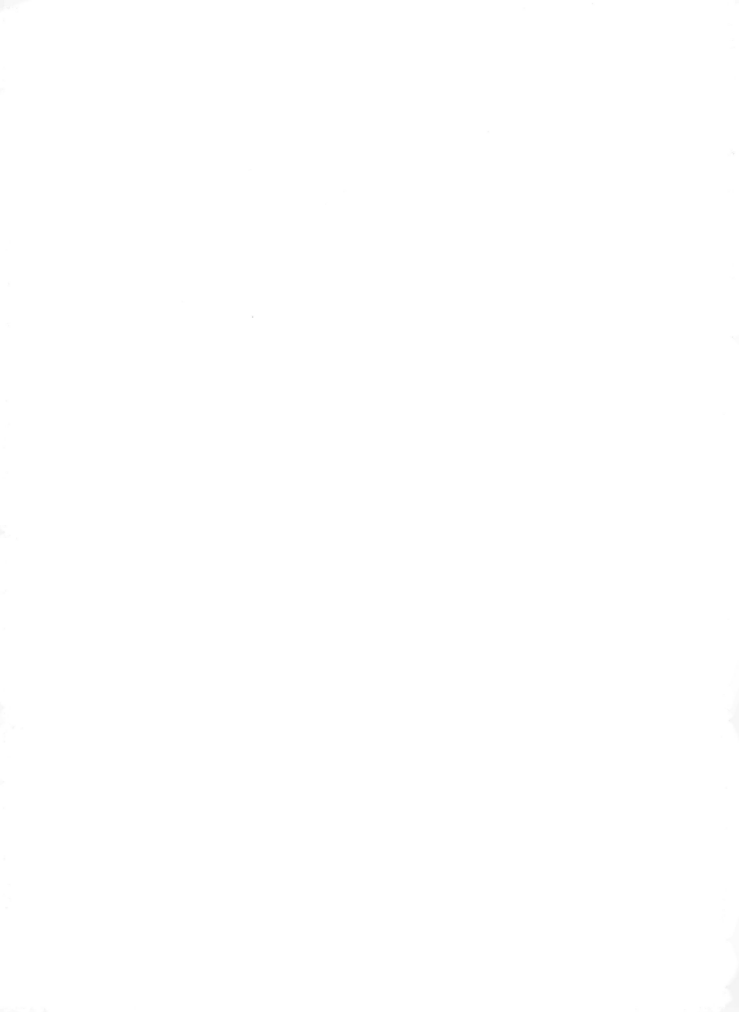

Parent–Child Questionnaire

Name of Child: _____ Today's Date: _____

Your Relationship to Child: _____

Directions. This questionnaire is about how you and your child have felt about each other in the past 2 WEEKS. For each question, circle the number that represents your choice. Please answer every item, and circle only one number for each item.

	Hardly at all 1	Not too much 2	Somewhat 3	Very much 4	Extremely much 5
1. How much do you and this child disagree and quarrel with each other?	1	2	3	4	5
2. How much do you order this child around?	1	2	3	4	5
3. How much do you and this child go places and do things together?	1	2	3	4	5
4. Some parents take away privileges a lot when their children misbehave, while other parents hardly ever take away privileges. How much do you take away privileges when this child misbehaves?	1	2	3	4	5
5. How much do you yell when this child misbehaves?	1	2	3	4	5
6. How much do you make this child feel ashamed or guilty for not doing what the child is supposed to do?	1	2	3	4	5
7. Some parents praise and compliment their children a lot, while other parents hardly ever praise and compliment their children. How much do you praise and compliment this child?	1	2	3	4	5
8. How much do you and this child get mad at and get in arguments with each other?	1	2	3	4	5

(continued)

Adapted and reprinted with permission of the developer (Wyndol Furman, University of Denver, 2022) in *Family–School Success for Children with ADHD: A Guide for Intervention* by Thomas J. Power, Jennifer A. Mautone, and Stephen L. Soffer (The Guilford Press, 2024). Permission to photocopy this material, or to download and print enlarged copies (*www.guilford.com/power2-forms*), is granted to purchasers of this book for personal use or use with students; see copyright page for details.

Parent–Child Questionnaire *(page 2 of 2)*

	Hardly at all 1	Not too much 2	Somewhat 3	Very much 4	Extremely much 5
9. How much do you lose your temper when this child misbehaves?	1	2	3	4	5
10. How much do you tell this child what to do?	1	2	3	4	5
11. How much do you tell this child that the child did a good job?	1	2	3	4	5
12. How much do you forbid this child from doing things the child likes when the child misbehaves?	1	2	3	4	5
13. How much do you nag or bug this child to do things?	1	2	3	4	5
14. How much do you play around and have fun with this child?	1	2	3	4	5
15. Some parents make their children feel bad about themselves a lot when they misbehave, while other parents do this a little. How much do you make this child feel bad when the child misbehaves?	1	2	3	4	5

Behavioral Health Checklist (Ages 4–7)

Please read each item and circle the word that tells how often your child has behaved like this in the past 4 weeks.

1. Feels sad	Never or rarely	Sometimes	Often	Very often
2. Shifts activities too quickly	Never or rarely	Sometimes	Often	Very often
3. Fights with other children	Never or rarely	Sometimes	Often	Very often
4. Has poor self-control	Never or rarely	Sometimes	Often	Very often
5. Is afraid of making mistakes	Never or rarely	Sometimes	Often	Very often
6. Is unable to slow down	Never or rarely	Sometimes	Often	Very often
7. Argues with adults	Never or rarely	Sometimes	Often	Very often
8. Worries	Never or rarely	Sometimes	Often	Very often
9. Is defiant	Never or rarely	Sometimes	Often	Very often
10. Can't sit still	Never or rarely	Sometimes	Often	Very often
11. Is easily annoyed or cranky	Never or rarely	Sometimes	Often	Very often
12. Refuses to share	Never or rarely	Sometimes	Often	Very often
13. Is too fearful	Never or rarely	Sometimes	Often	Very often
14. Has trouble paying attention	Never or rarely	Sometimes	Often	Very often
15. Is unhappy	Never or rarely	Sometimes	Often	Very often
16. Is disobedient	Never or rarely	Sometimes	Often	Very often
17. Argues with peers	Never or rarely	Sometimes	Often	Very often
18. Can't concentrate	Never or rarely	Sometimes	Often	Very often
19. Gets along with peers	Never or rarely	Sometimes	Often	Very often
20. Relates well with parents	Never or rarely	Sometimes	Often	Very often
21. Has self-control	Never or rarely	Sometimes	Often	Very often
22. Relates well with teachers	Never or rarely	Sometimes	Often	Very often

---

Copyright © 2013 Children's Hospital of Philadelphia. Adapted and reprinted with permission in *Family–School Success for Children with ADHD: A Guide for Intervention* by Thomas J. Power, Jennifer A. Mautone, and Stephen L. Soffer (The Guilford Press, 2024). Permission to photocopy this material, or to download and print additional copies (*www.guilford.com/power2-forms*), is granted to purchasers of this book for personal use or use with students; see copyright page for details.

Behavioral Health Checklist (Ages 8–12)

Please read each item and circle the word that tells how often your child has behaved like this in the past 4 weeks.

1. Feels hopeless	Never or rarely	Sometimes	Often	Very often
2. Has difficulty sustaining attention	Never or rarely	Sometimes	Often	Very often
3. Fights with other children	Never or rarely	Sometimes	Often	Very often
4. Talks excessively	Never or rarely	Sometimes	Often	Very often
5. Is afraid of making mistakes	Never or rarely	Sometimes	Often	Very often
6. Has difficulty awaiting turn	Never or rarely	Sometimes	Often	Very often
7. Is down on self	Never or rarely	Sometimes	Often	Very often
8. Steals	Never or rarely	Sometimes	Often	Very often
9. Worries	Never or rarely	Sometimes	Often	Very often
10. Fidgets or squirms in seat	Never or rarely	Sometimes	Often	Very often
11. Feels sad	Never or rarely	Sometimes	Often	Very often
12. Teases others	Never or rarely	Sometimes	Often	Very often
13. Loses temper too easily	Never or rarely	Sometimes	Often	Very often
14. Avoids tasks that require effort	Never or rarely	Sometimes	Often	Very often
15. Breaks the rules	Never or rarely	Sometimes	Often	Very often
16. Loses things necessary for activities	Never or rarely	Sometimes	Often	Very often
17. Is too fearful	Never or rarely	Sometimes	Often	Very often
18. Lies or cheats	Never or rarely	Sometimes	Often	Very often
19. Gets along with peers	Never or rarely	Sometimes	Often	Very often
20. Relates well with parents	Never or rarely	Sometimes	Often	Very often
21. Has self-control	Never or rarely	Sometimes	Often	Very often
22. Relates well with teachers	Never or rarely	Sometimes	Often	Very often

---

Copyright © 2013 Children's Hospital of Philadelphia. Adapted and reprinted with permission in *Family–School Success for Children with ADHD: A Guide for Intervention* by Thomas J. Power, Jennifer A. Mautone, and Stephen L. Soffer (The Guilford Press, 2024). Permission to photocopy this material, or to download and print additional copies (*www.guilford.com/power2-forms*), is granted to purchasers of this book for personal use or use with students; see copyright page for details.

Homework Performance Questionnaire (for Parents)

Child's name: _____ Grade Level: _____ Today's Date: _____

Parent's name: _____ Your Relationship to Child: _____

Part A. Please complete the following questions. The word *homework* refers to academic tasks assigned by teachers for students to complete at home, in after-school programs, or in school when students are not receiving instruction.

1. What is the average amount of time your child spends doing homework each day?
   - ____ 15 minutes or less
   - ____ 30 minutes
   - ____ 45 minutes
   - ____ 1 hour
   - ____ 1 hour and 30 minutes
   - ____ 2 hours
   - ____ 2 hours and 30 minutes
   - ____ 3 hours
   - ____ More than 3 hours

2. Is your child having trouble completing homework in any subjects   ____ Yes   ____ No
   If yes, indicate which subjects: _____

3. Do the teachers expect your child to write homework assignments in a notebook?
   ____ Yes   ____ No

4. If your child can't remember what to do for homework, what do you do? Check all that apply.
   - ____ Have my child call a friend
   - ____ Return to the school at the end of the day to get the homework
   - ____ Check the school or teacher website that posts homework assignments
   - ____ Call the homework hotline
   - ____ Nothing. We just do the best we can.
   - ____ Other _____
   - ____ Not appropriate—my child always remembers what to do for homework

Part B. For the items below, circle the answer that tells how often each behavior has happened **DURING THE PAST 4 WEEKS.** Please answer each item.

5. My child must be reminded to begin homework.
   rarely/never   some of the time   most of the time   always/almost always

6. My child is able to complete math homework without help.
   rarely/never   some of the time   most of the time   always/almost always

7. The teachers understand how homework can affect family life.
   rarely/never   some of the time   most of the time   always/almost always

8. My child needs close supervision to get homework done.
   rarely/never   some of the time   most of the time   always/almost always

(continued)

Copyright © 2008 Children's Hospital of Philadelphia. Reprinted with permission in *Family–School Success for Children with ADHD: A Guide for Intervention* by Thomas J. Power, Jennifer A. Mautone, and Stephen L. Soffer (The Guilford Press, 2024). Permission to photocopy this material, or to download and print additional copies (*www.guilford.com/power2-forms*), is granted to purchasers of this book for personal use or use with students; see copyright page for details.

Homework Performance Questionnaire (for Parents) *(page 2 of 2)*

9. My child understands how to do the homework assigned by the teacher.
   rarely/never   some of the time   most of the time   always/almost always
10. The teachers communicate effectively with our family about homework.
    rarely/never   some of the time   most of the time   always/almost always
11. My child wastes time during homework.
    rarely/never   some of the time   most of the time   always/almost always
12. Homework assignments are easy for my child to complete.
    rarely/never   some of the time   most of the time   always/almost always
13. My child is ready to start homework when it's time to begin.
    rarely/never   some of the time   most of the time   always/almost always
14. The teachers seem willing to help if we have homework problems.
    rarely/never   some of the time   most of the time   always/almost always
15. My child is able to complete reading and language arts homework without help.
    rarely/never   some of the time   most of the time   always/almost always
16. Once started, my child works steadily on homework.
    rarely/never   some of the time   most of the time   always/almost always
17. The teachers assign too much homework.
    rarely/never   some of the time   most of the time   always/almost always
18. Homework assignments are too difficult for my child.
    rarely/never   some of the time   most of the time   always/almost always
19. The teachers and I have similar ideas about homework.
    rarely/never   some of the time   most of the time   always/almost always
20. My child tries to avoid doing homework.
    rarely/never   some of the time   most of the time   always/almost always
21. The teachers' homework assignments are confusing to me.
    rarely/never   some of the time   most of the time   always/almost always
22. My child needs help to understand how to complete homework assignments.
    rarely/never   some of the time   most of the time   always/almost always
23. My child brings home the books and materials needed to complete homework.
    rarely/never   some of the time   most of the time   always/almost always
24. The teachers seem interested in helping my child complete homework assignments.
    rarely/never   some of the time   most of the time   always/almost always
25. My child gets confused when doing homework.
    rarely/never   some of the time   most of the time   always/almost always
26. My child takes completed homework back to class.
    rarely/never   some of the time   most of the time   always/almost always
27. My child follows my directions when doing homework.
    rarely/never   some of the time   most of the time   always/almost always

Cuestionario Sobre Desempeño en las Tareas/Asignaciones (para Padres)

Nombre del niño/a: _____ Grado escolar: _____ Fecha de hoy: _____

Nombre del padre/madre: _____ Su parentesco con el niño/a: _____

Sección A. Complete las siguientes preguntas. (Las palabras "asignación" o "asignaciones" se refieren a tareas académicas asignadas por maestros para que sean completadas en la casa, en programas después de clase, o en la escuela cuando los estudiantes no están recibiendo instrucción)

1. En promedio, ¿cuánto tiempo dedica su hijo/a a hacer las asignaciones cada día?

   ____ 15 minutos o menos   ____ 2 horas
   ____ 30 minutos   ____ 2 horas y 30 minutos
   ____ 45 minutos   ____ 3 horas
   ____ 1 hora   ____ Más de 3 horas
   ____ 1 hora y 30 minutos

2. ¿Su hijo/a tiene dificultades para completar la asignación de alguna materia (asignatura)?
   ____ Sí ____ No

   En caso afirmativo, indique las asignaturas: _____

3. ¿Los maestros esperan que su hijo/a escriba las asignaciones en un cuaderno (una libreta)?
   ____ Sí ____ No

4. Si su hijo/a no puede recordar las asignaciones qué debía completar, ¿usted qué hace? Marque todas las opciones que correspondan.

   ____ Hago que mi hijo/a llame por teléfono a un amigo
   ____ Regreso a la escuela al finalizar el día escolar para conseguir las asignaciones.
   ____ Visito el sitio Web de la escuela o del maestro/a donde se publican las tareas
   ____ Llamo por teléfono a la línea directa de asistencia con las asignaciones.
   ____ Nada. Hacemos lo mejor que podemos.
   ____ Otro _____
   ____ No corresponde—mi hijo/a siempre recuerda las asignaciones que debe hacer (completar)

Sección B. Para las frases siguientes, marque con un círculo la respuesta que indica la frecuencia con la que ha sucedido cada comportamiento EN LAS ÚLTIMAS 4 SEMANAS Por favor responda a todas las frases.

5. A mi hijo/a hay que recordarle que comience a hacer las asignaciones.

   casi nunca/nunca   a veces   la mayoría de las veces   siempre/casi siempre

6. Mi hijo/a puede completar la asignación de matemática sin ayuda.

   casi nunca/nunca   a veces   la mayoría de las veces   siempre/casi siempre

7. Los maestros/as comprenden cómo las asignaciones puede afectar la vida familiar.

   casi nunca/nunca   a veces   la mayoría de las veces   siempre/casi siempre

(continuado)

Cuestionario Sobre Desempeño en las Tareas/Asignaciones *(página 2 de 2)*

8. Es necesario supervisar de cerca de mi hijo/a para que complete las asignaciones.
   casi nunca/nunca   a veces   la mayoría de las veces   siempre/casi siempre

9. Mi hijo/a entiende cómo completar las asignaciones que da el maestro/a.
   casi nunca/nunca   a veces   la mayoría de las veces   siempre/casi siempre

10. Los maestros/as se comunican de forma eficaz con nuestra familia sobre las asignaciones.
    casi nunca/nunca   a veces   la mayoría de las veces   siempre/casi siempre

11. Mi hijo/a pierde el tiempo mientras hace las asignaciones.
    casi nunca/nunca   a veces   la mayoría de las veces   siempre/casi siempre

12. A mi hijo/a le resulta fácil completar las asignaciones.
    casi nunca/nunca   a veces   la mayoría de las veces   siempre/casi siempre

13. Mi hijo/a se muestra dispuesto/a para comenzar las asignaciones cuando llega el momento de hacerlas.
    casi nunca/nunca   a veces   la mayoría de las veces   siempre/casi siempre

14. Los maestros/as muestran voluntad de ayudar si tenemos problemas con las asignaciones.
    casi nunca/nunca   a veces   la mayoría de las veces   siempre/casi siempre

15. Mi hijo/a puede completar las asignaciones de lectura y gramática sin ayuda.
    casi nunca/nunca   a veces   la mayoría de las veces   siempre/casi siempre

16. Una vez que comienza, mi hijo/a hace las asignaciones a un ritmo constante.
    casi nunca/nunca   a veces   la mayoría de las veces   siempre/casi siempre

17. Los maestros/as dan demasiadas asignaciones.
    casi nunca/nunca   a veces   la mayoría de las veces   siempre/casi siempre

18. Las asignaciones son demasiado difíciles para mi hijo.
    casi nunca/nunca   a veces   la mayoría de las veces   siempre/casi siempre

19. Los maestros/as y yo tenemos opiniones similares respecto a las asignaciones.
    casi nunca/nunca   a veces   la mayoría de las veces   siempre/casi siempre

20. Mi hijo/a trata de evitar hacer las asignaciones.
    casi nunca/nunca   a veces   la mayoría de las veces   siempre/casi siempre

21. Las asignaciones que dan los maestros/as me resultan difíciles de entender.
    casi nunca/nunca   a veces   la mayoría de las veces   siempre/casi siempre

22. Mi hijo/a necesita ayuda para entender cómo debe completar las asignaciones.
    casi nunca/nunca   a veces   la mayoría de las veces   siempre/casi siempre

23. Mi hijo/a trae a casa los libros y materiales necesarios para completar las asignaciones.
    casi nunca/nunca   a veces   la mayoría de las veces   siempre/casi siempre

24. Los maestros/as parecen interesados/as en ayudar a mi hijo/a a completar las asignaciones.
    casi nunca/nunca   a veces   la mayoría de las veces   siempre/casi siempre

25. Mi hijo/a se confunde cuando hace las asignaciones.
    casi nunca/nunca   a veces   la mayoría de las veces   siempre/casi siempre

26. Mi hijo/a va a clase con las asignaciones hechas.
    casi nunca/nunca   a veces   la mayoría de las veces   siempre/casi siempre

27. Mi hijo/a cumple mis indicaciones cuando hace las asignaciones.
    casi nunca/nunca   a veces   la mayoría de las veces   siempre/casi siempre

Homework Performance Questionnaire (for Teachers)

Student's name: _____ Date: _____

Is the child classified as a special education student? (yes or no) _____

Teacher's name: _____ Grade level: _____

Part A. Please complete the following questions.

1. Please indicate which subjects you teach this child. Select all that apply.
   - ____ Reading
   - ____ Language Arts (including Spelling)
   - ____ Social Studies
   - ____ Math
   - ____ Science
   - ____ Other _____

2. What is the maximum amount of time that students in this grade should be spending each day doing homework (including all subjects)? Select only one.
   - ____ 15 minutes or less
   - ____ 30 minutes
   - ____ 45 minutes
   - ____ 1 hour
   - ____ 1 hour and 30 minutes
   - ____ 2 hours
   - ____ 2 hours and 30 minutes
   - ____ 3 hours
   - ____ More than 3 hours

3. Is this student expected to write homework assignments in a notebook? ____ Yes ____ No

4. How often do you check to see that this student writes down homework assignments accurately? Select only one.
   - ____ Never or rarely
   - ____ Less than once per week
   - ____ Once per week
   - ____ Once or twice a week
   - ____ 3 to 4 times per week
   - ____ Every day

5. How often do you check to see that this student takes home the books and materials needed for homework? Select only one.
   - ____ Never or rarely
   - ____ Less than once per week
   - ____ Once per week
   - ____ Once or twice per week
   - ____ 3 to 4 times per week
   - ____ Every day

6. What do you recommend to families with a child who has trouble remembering what to do for homework and writing down assignments? Select all that apply.
   - ____ Use a homework assignment book that is checked by parents and teachers
   - ____ Contact a classmate
   - ____ Check the school website that posts homework assignments
   - ____ Call the homework hotline
   - ____ Parents should write a note on days there is a problem

(continued)

Copyright © 2008 Children's Hospital of Philadelphia. Reprinted with permission in *Family–School Success for Children with ADHD: A Guide for Intervention* by Thomas J. Power, Jennifer A. Mautone, and Stephen L. Soffer (The Guilford Press, 2024). Permission to photocopy this material, or to download and print additional copies (*www.guilford.com/power2-forms*), is granted to purchasers of this book for personal use or use with students; see copyright page for details.

Homework Performance Questionnaire (for Teachers) *(page 2 of 3)*

____ Nothing. Family should do the best they can.
____ Other _____

7. How often do you check to see that homework has been completed accurately? Select only one.
   ____ Never or rarely   ____ Once or twice per week
   ____ Less than once per week   ____ 3 to 4 times per week
   ____ Once per week   ____ Every day

8. What percentage of the child's grade is determined by the amount or quality of homework completed? Select only one.
   ____ 0%   ____ 21 to 30%
   ____ 1 to 5%   ____ 31 to 40%
   ____ 6 to 10%   ____ 41 to 50%
   ____ 11 to 20%   ____ More than 50%

Part B. For items 9 through 23, select the response that indicates the amount or percentage of the time that each behavior has occurred DURING THE PAST 4 WEEKS. Please complete each item.

9. This student finishes homework assignments (regardless of quality).

Never/rarely	seldom	not often	some of the time	often	usually	almost always/always
0–10%	11–20%	21–40%	41–60%	61–80%	81–90%	91–100%

10. This student has shown the ability to complete homework assignments independently.

Never/rarely	seldom	not often	some of the time	often	usually	almost always/always
0–10%	11–20%	21–40%	41–60%	61–80%	81–90%	91–100%

11. This student turns in homework on time.

Never/rarely	seldom	not often	some of the time	often	usually	almost always/always
0–10%	11–20%	21–40%	41–60%	61–80%	81–90%	91–100%

12. This student seems to manage time effectively during homework.

Never/rarely	seldom	not often	some of the time	often	usually	almost always/always
0–10%	11–20%	21–40%	41–60%	61–80%	81–90%	91–100%

13. Forms and tests are signed and returned to me on time.

Never/rarely	seldom	not often	some of the time	often	usually	almost always/always
0–10%	11–20%	21–40%	41–60%	61–80%	81–90%	91–100%

14. Homework assignments are easy for this child to complete.

Never/rarely	seldom	not often	some of the time	often	usually	almost always/always
0–10%	11–20%	21–40%	41–60%	61–80%	81–90%	91–100%

15. This student turns in homework that is messy.

Never/rarely	seldom	not often	some of the time	often	usually	almost always/always
0–10%	11–20%	21–40%	41–60%	61–80%	81–90%	91–100%

16. As far as I know, this student understands how to do homework assignments upon leaving my class each day.

Never/rarely	seldom	not often	some of the time	often	usually	almost always/always
0–10%	11–20%	21–40%	41–60%	61–80%	81–90%	91–100%

17. This student organizes materials needed for homework before leaving class.

Never/rarely	seldom	not often	some of the time	often	usually	almost always/always
0–10%	11–20%	21–40%	41–60%	61–80%	81–90%	91–100%

(continued)

Homework Performance Questionnaire (for Teachers) *(page 3 of 3)*

18. This student needs help to understand how to complete homework assignments.

Never/rarely	seldom	not often	some of the time	often	usually	almost always/always
0–10%	11–20%	21–40%	41–60%	61–80%	81–90%	91–100%

19. By the end of class, this student knows how to do the assignments given for homework.

Never/rarely	seldom	not often	some of the time	often	usually	almost always/always
0–10%	11–20%	21–40%	41–60%	61–80%	81–90%	91–100%

20. This student turns in homework that is completed accurately.

Never/rarely	seldom	not often	some of the time	often	usually	almost always/always
0–10%	11–20%	21–40%	41–60%	61–80%	81–90%	91–100%

21. This student makes an effort to complete homework.

Never/rarely	seldom	not often	some of the time	often	usually	almost always/always
0–10%	11–20%	21–40%	41–60%	61–80%	81–90%	91–100%

22. Homework assignments seem to be too difficult for this child.

Never/rarely	seldom	not often	some of the time	often	usually	almost always/always
0–10%	11–20%	21–40%	41–60%	61–80%	81–90%	91–100%

23. At the end of class, I am confident this student can do the homework assigned.

Never/rarely	seldom	not often	some of the time	often	usually	almost always/always
0–10%	11–20%	21–40%	41–60%	61–80%	81–90%	91–100%

Part C. For items 24 and 25, select the percentage that best describes the child's performance DURING THE PAST 4 WEEKS. Please complete each item.

24. Estimate the percentage of homework completed (regardless of accuracy).

0–10%	11–20%	21–40%	41–60%	61–80%	81–90%	91–100%

25. Estimate the percentage of homework that this child is able to complete correctly without assistance.

0–10%	11–20%	21–40%	41–60%	61–80%	81–90%	91–100%

Part D. Please provide additional comments about this student's homework performance. Also, comment on any factors that influence this student's homework performance.

Academic Proficiency Scale (APS)

Student Name: _____ Date: _____

School: _____ Grade: _____

INSTRUCTIONS:

For each school subject listed below, please ✓ to indicate the child's performance **compared to the standard that you would expect at this time of year.** Please choose only ONE option for each subject. If the child does NOT have a subject please ✓ Not applicable.

Reading	☐ Well below	☐ Below	☐ At the standard	☐ Above	☐ Well above	☐ Not applicable
Spelling	☐ Well below	☐ Below	☐ At the standard	☐ Above	☐ Well above	☐ Not applicable
Language Arts	☐ Well below	☐ Below	☐ At the standard	☐ Above	☐ Well above	☐ Not applicable
Social Studies	☐ Well below	☐ Below	☐ At the standard	☐ Above	☐ Well above	☐ Not applicable
Science	☐ Well below	☐ Below	☐ At the standard	☐ Above	☐ Well above	☐ Not applicable
Math	☐ Well below	☐ Below	☐ At the standard	☐ Above	☐ Well above	☐ Not applicable

---

Adapted and reprinted with permission of the developers (Howard Abikoff and Richard Gallagher) in *Family–School Success for Children with ADHD: A Guide for Intervention* by Thomas J. Power, Jennifer A. Mautone, and Stephen L. Soffer. (The Guilford Press, 2024). Permission to photocopy this material, or to download and print additional copies (*www.guilford.com/power2-forms*), is granted to purchasers of this book for personal use or use with students; see copyright page for details.

Family–School Success Program Evaluation Scale

Date: _____

Section A. Please rate how helpful each part of the program has been for you and your family.

1. Strategies to strengthen the parent–child relationship (special time, catch child being good).

1	2	3	4
Not very helpful	Somewhat helpful	Helpful	Very helpful

2. Learning about and applying the A-B-C model (antecedents, behavior, consequences).

1	2	3	4
Not very helpful	Somewhat helpful	Helpful	Very helpful

3. Strategies to help your child with homework.

1	2	3	4
Not very helpful	Somewhat helpful	Helpful	Very helpful

4. Strategies to help your child in school (e.g., collaborating with teacher, daily report card).

1	2	3	4
Not very helpful	Somewhat helpful	Helpful	Very helpful

5. Using punishment strategies successfully.

1	2	3	4
Not very helpful	Somewhat helpful	Helpful	Very helpful

6. Developing strategies to manage your emotions and take care of yourself as a parent.

1	2	3	4
Not very helpful	Somewhat helpful	Helpful	Very helpful

Section B. Please rate how helpful each aspect of the program has been for your family.

7. Telephone calls with a group leader between sessions.

1	2	3	4
Not very helpful	Somewhat helpful	Helpful	Very helpful

8. Telephone calls to your child's teacher/school staff.

1	2	3	4
Not very helpful	Somewhat helpful	Helpful	Very helpful

9. The handouts.

1	2	3	4
Not very helpful	Somewhat helpful	Helpful	Very helpful

(continued)

Copyright © 2002 Children's Hospital of Philadelphia. Reprinted with permission in *Family–School Success for Children with ADHD: A Guide for Intervention* by Thomas J. Power, Jennifer A. Mautone, and Stephen L. Soffer (The Guilford Press, 2024). Permission to photocopy this material, or to download and print additional copies (*www.guilford.com/power2-forms*), is granted to purchasers of this book for personal use or use with students; see copyright page for details.

Family–School Success Program Evaluation Scale *(page 2 of 2)*

10. The parent homework assignments.

1	2	3	4
Not very helpful	Somewhat helpful	Helpful	Very helpful

11. The opportunity to share experiences with and learn from other parents.

1	2	3	4
Not very helpful	Somewhat helpful	Helpful	Very helpful

Section C. Please rate the extent to which you agree with the following items.

12. The sessions were well organized.

1	2	3	4
Disagree	Somewhat disagree	Somewhat agree	Agree

13. The clinician(s) did a good job managing time during the group sessions.

1	2	3	4
Disagree	Somewhat disagree	Somewhat agree	Agree

14. The clinician(s) showed respect for my family.

1	2	3	4
Disagree	Somewhat disagree	Somewhat agree	Agree

15. I was able to build trust in the clinician(s).

1	2	3	4
Disagree	Somewhat disagree	Somewhat agree	Agree

16. The clinician(s) has been helpful to my family.

1	2	3	4
Disagree	Somewhat disagree	Somewhat agree	Agree

17. The clinician(s) understands our family situation.

1	2	3	4
Disagree	Somewhat disagree	Somewhat agree	Agree

Section D. Please provide other feedback/comments.

18. What aspects of the program have been the most helpful to you?

19. What suggestions do you have for us that may be helpful for future groups?

Thank you very much for taking the time to provide our team with this feedback.

Coding Manual for Family–School Success Between-Session Homework Assignments

Instructions:

- Homework Codes
  - 2 = Complete
  - 1 = Attempted
  - 0 = Not attempted at all or missing
- The Session # is the number of the session in which homework was assigned to the families. For example, homework assigned during Session 1 was the "Noticing Positive/Desired Behavior" worksheet, and it is labeled at the top of the worksheet as "Session 1."
- Attendance
  - Y = Parents attended the session when the homework was assigned
  - N = Parents did not attend the session when homework was assigned, or parents made up the session on the same day as their next session (i.e., they had no time to complete homework before their next session)
- Calculate the following scores:
  - Total homework score for the full program = credit for homework completed divided by total possible homework score (22)
  - Adjusted homework score = credit for homework completed divided by total possible homework score only for homework assigned when parents attended a session

Session #	Worksheet Title	Therapist Instructions to Parent	Scoring Instructions
1	Noticing Positive/Desired Behavior	Record positive behaviors, indicate parent response, and indicate child response	2 = recorded at least 2 positive behaviors, positive reinforcers, AND child responses 1 = filled in some of the worksheet
2	Child's Game	Record occasions during which they engaged in the Child's Game (date, time, activity, and child response)	2 = recorded at least 2 occasions participated in Child's Game (including activity and child response) 1 = filled in some of the worksheet
3	A-B-C Worksheet	Complete A-B-C analysis of 1 or 2 problem behaviors during the week (recorded antecedent, behavior, consequences, and outcome)	2 = completed ABC + outcome for at least 1 behavior 1 = filled in some of the worksheet
3	Reward Menu	Develop a menu of reinforcers (rewards)	2 = listed at least 3 reinforcers 1 = listed less than 3 reinforcers

(continued)

Copyright © 2022 Children's Hospital of Philadelphia. Reprinted with permission in *Family–School Success for Children with ADHD: A Guide for Intervention* by Thomas J. Power, Jennifer A. Mautone, and Stephen L. Soffer (The Guilford Press, 2024). Permission to photocopy this material, or to download and print additional copies (*www.guilford.com/power2-forms*), is granted to purchasers of this book for personal use or use with students; see copyright page for details.

Coding Manual for Family–School Success
Between-Session Homework Assignments *(page 2 of 3)*

Session #	Worksheet Title	Therapist Instructions to Parent	Scoring Instructions
4	Daily Report Card (DRC)	Develop a DRC with target behaviors	2 = DRC with at least 2 target behaviors indicated 1 = DRC with less than 2 target behaviors indicated
5	Target Behaviors	List possible target behaviors (stated positively) and circle the 2–3 behaviors to focus on *Note:* Do not penalize for not completing difficulty section of version of form handed out at Session 4	2 = at least 2 target behaviors listed 1 = 1 target behavior listed
5	Home Rewards Worksheet (setting up a token economy)	Complete Home Rewards Worksheet	2 = completed Home Rewards Worksheet for at least 2 target behaviors 1 = incomplete worksheet
6	Homework A-B-C Worksheet	Identify problematic homework behaviors and complete the Homework A-B-C Worksheet for each (ABC + Outcomes)	2 = recorded at least 2 instances (i.e., could be same behavior on different occasions or 2 different behaviors) 1 = recorded 1 or fewer instances of homework ABC
6	Homework Ritual Worksheet	Summarize Where, When, and What of homework ritual using worksheet	2 = described Where, When and What (don't need checkmarks if clearly described) 1 = made checkmarks only and/or did not complete all 3 sections
7	Goal-Setting Tool or Summary Sheet	Complete Goal-Setting Tool or Goal-Setting Summary Sheet	2 = any complete Goal-Setting Tool or Goal-Setting Summary Sheet (all lines filled out) 1 = incomplete forms
8	Using Punishment Strategically	Identify target behaviors and identify what the punishment will be	2 = listed 1 target behavior that also has a punishment with it 1 = listed only a behavior or only a punishment

(continued)

Coding Manual for Family–School Success Between-Session Homework Assignments (page 3 of 3)

Scoring Sheet for Family–School Success Between Session Homework Assignments

Family Name/Child ID#: _____

Coder: _____

Session #	Worksheet Title	Homework Code	Attendance	Assigned
1	Noticing Positive/Desired Behavior	0 1 2	Y / N	Y / N
2	Child's Game	0 1 2	Y / N	Y / N
3	A-B-C Worksheet	0 1 2	Y / N	Y / N
3	Reward List	0 1 2	Y / N	Y / N
4	Home–school note	0 1 2	Y / N	Y / N
5	Target Behaviors	0 1 2	Y / N	Y / N
5	Setting up token economy checklist	0 1 2	Y / N	Y / N
6	Homework ABC	0 1 2	Y / N	Y / N
6	Homework Ritual Worksheet	0 1 2	Y / N	Y / N
7	Goal Setting Tool or Summary Sheet	0 1 2	Y / N	Y / N
8	Using Punishment Successfully	0 1 2	Y / N	Y / N

Scoring Key for Measures

Parent–Child Questionnaire	
Subscale	Items
Negative/Ineffective Parenting	1, 2, 4, 5, 6, 8, 9, 10, 12, 13, 15
Positive Parenting	3, 7, 11, 14
Note: No items are reverse scored.	

Behavioral Health Checklist (Ages 4–7)	
Subscale	Items
Internalizing	1, 5, 8, 11, 13, 15
Externalizing	3, 7, 9, 12, 16, 17
ADHD	2, 4, 6, 10, 14, 18
Strengths	19, 20, 21, 22
Note: No items are reverse scored.	

Behavioral Health Checklist (Ages 8–12)	
Subscale	Items
Internalizing	1, 5, 7, 9, 11, 17
Externalizing	3, 8, 12, 13, 15, 18
ADHD	2, 4, 6, 10, 14, 16
Strengths	19, 20, 21, 22
Note: No items are reverse scored.	

Homework Performance Questionnaire (for Parents) (English and Spanish Versions)	
Subscale	Items
Child Self-Regulation	5, 8, 11, 13, 16, 20, 23, 26, 27
Child Competence	6, 9, 12, 15, 18, 22, 25
Teacher Support	7, 10, 14, 17, 19, 21, 24
Note: Items 5, 8, 11, 17, 18, 20, 21, 22, and 25 are reverse scored.	

Homework Performance Questionnaire (for Teachers)	
Subscale	Items
Child Self-Regulation	9, 11, 12, 13, 15, 17, 20, 21, 24
Child Competence	10, 14, 16, 18, 19, 22, 23, 25
Note: Items 15, 18, and 22 are reverse scored.	

Academic Proficiency Scale (APS)
Items are scored: 0 = well below standard; 1 = below standard; 2 = at the standard; 3 = above standard; 4 = well above standard. Average item score is the sum of all scores divided by the number of items rated.

Family–School Success Program Evaluation Scale	
Sections	Items
Perception of Program Content	1, 2, 3, 4, 5, 6
Perception of Implementation Supports	7, 8, 9, 10, 11
Perception of Clinician Effectiveness	12, 13, 14, 15, 16, 17
Note: No items are reverse scored.	

References

Abikoff, H., Gallagher, R., Wells, K. C., Murray, D. W., Huang, L., & Petkova E. (2013). Remediating organizational functioning in children with ADHD: Immediate and long-term effects from a randomized controlled trial. *Journal of Consulting and Clinical Psychology, 81*, 113–128.

Adams, E. L., Smith, D., Caccavale, L. J., & Bean, M. K. (2021). Parents are stressed! Patterns of parent stress across COVID-19. *Frontiers in Psychiatry, 12*, 626456.

Ambrosini, P. J. (2000). Historical development and present status of the Schedule for Affective Disorders and Schizophrenia for School-Age Children (K-SADS). *Journal of the American Academy of Child & Adolescent Psychiatry, 39*, 49–58.

Anderson, K. J., & Minke, K. M. (2007). Parent involvement in education: Toward an understanding of parents' decision making. *Journal of Educational Research, 100*, 311–323.

Anesko, K. M., Schoiock, G., Ramirez, R., & Levine, F. M. (1987). The Homework Problem Checklist: Assessing children's homework difficulties. *Behavioral Assessment, 9*, 179–185.

Asarnow, J. R., Kolko, D. J., Miranda, J., & Kazak, A. E. (2017). The Pediatric Patient-Centered Medical Home: Innovative models for improving behavioral health. *American Psychologist, 72*(1), 13–27.

Asarnow, J. R., Rozenman, M., Wiblin, J., & Zeltzer, L. (2015). Integrated medical-behavioral care compared with usual primary care for child and adolescent behavioral health: A meta-analysis. *JAMA Pediatrics, 169*(10), 929–937.

Bandura, A. (1971). *Social learning theory*. New York: General Learning Press.

Bandura, A. (1977). *Social learning theory*. Oxford, UK: Prentice-Hall.

Barbaresi, W. J., Campbell, L., Diekroger, E. A., Froehlich, T. E., Liu, Y. H., O'Malley, E., et al. (2020a). Society for Developmental and Behavioral Pediatrics clinical practice guideline for the assessment and treatment of children and adolescents with complex attention-deficit/hyperactivity disorder. *Journal of Developmental and Behavioral Pediatrics, 41*, S535–S557.

Barbaresi, W. J., Campbell, L., Diekroger, E. A., Froehlich, T. E., Liu, Y. H., O'Malley, E., et al. (2020b). Society for Developmental and Behavioral Pediatrics clinical practice guideline for the assessment and treatment of children and adolescents with complex attention-deficit/hyperactivity disorder: Process of care algorithms. *Journal of Developmental and Behavioral Pediatrics, 41*, S558–S574.

Baydar, N., Reid, M. J., & Webster-Stratton, C. (2003). The role of mental health factors and program engagement in the effectiveness of a preventive parenting program for Head Start Mothers. *Child Development, 74*, 1433–1453.

Bikic, A., Reichow, B., McCauley, S. A., Ibrahim, K., & Sukhodolsky, D. G. (2017). Meta-analysis of organizational skills interventions for children and adolescents with attention deficit/hyperactivity disorder. *Clinical Psychology Review, 52*, 108–123.

Booster, G., Mautone, J. A., Nissley-Tsiopinis, J., Van Dyke, D., & Power, T. J. (2016). Reductions in negative parenting practices mediate the effect of a family–school intervention for children with ADHD. *School Psychology Review, 45,* 192–208.

Bronfenbrenner, U. (2009). *The ecology of human development: Experiments by nature and design.* Cambridge, MA: Harvard University Press.

Chacko, A., Wymbs, B. T., Arnold, F. W., Pelham, W. E., Swanger-Gagne, M., Girio, E. L., et al. (2009). Enhancing traditional behavioral parent training for single mothers of children with ADHD. *Journal of Clinical Child and Adolescent Psychology, 38,* 206–218.

Christenson, S. L., & Sheridan, S. M. (2001). *Schools and families: Creating essential connections for learning.* New York: Guilford Press.

Chronis, A. M., Fabiano, G. A., Gnagy, E. M., Onyango, A. N., Pelham, W. E., Williams, A., et al. (2004). An evaluation of the Summer Treatment Program for children with attention-deficit/hyperactivity disorder using a treatment withdrawal design. *Behavior Therapy, 35,* 561–585.

Chronis-Tuscano, A., O'Brien, K., & Danko, C. M. (2020). *Supporting caregivers of children with ADHD: An integrated parenting program (therapist's guide).* New York: Oxford University Press.

Chronis-Tuscano, A., Wang, C. H., Woods, K. E., Strickland, J., & Stein, M. A. (2017). Parent ADHD and evidence-based treatment for their children: Review and directions for future research. *Journal of Abnormal Child Psychology, 45,* 501–517.

Clarke, A. T., Marshall, S. A., Mautone, J. A., Soffer, S. L., Jones, H. A., Costigan, T. E., et al. (2015). Parent attendance and homework adherence predict response to a family–school intervention for children with ADHD. *Journal of Clinical Child and Adolescent Psychology, 44,* 58–67.

Conners, C. K., Epstein, J. N., March, J. S., Angold, A., Wells, K. C., Klaric, J., et al. (2001). Multimodal treatment of ADHD in the MTA: An alternative outcome analysis. *Journal of the American Academy of Child and Adolescent Psychiatry, 40,* 159–167.

Danielson, M. L., Bitsko, R. H., Ghandour, R. M., Holbrook, J. R., Kogan, M. D., & Blumberg, S. J. (2018). Prevalence of parent-reported ADHD diagnosis and associated treatment among U.S. children and adolescents. *Journal of Clinical Child and Adolescent Psychology, 47,* 199–212.

Dawson, A. E., Wymbs, B. T., Marshall, S. A., Mautone, J. A., & Power, T. J. (2016). The role of parental ADHD in sustaining the effects of a family-school intervention for ADHD. *Journal of Clinical Child and Adolescent Psychology, 45,* 305–319.

Deci, E. L., & Ryan, R. M. (1985). *Intrinsic motivation and self-determination in human behavior.* New York: Plenum Press.

DuPaul, G. J., & Power, T. J. (2008). Improving school outcomes for students with ADHD: Using the right strategies in the context of the right relationships. *Journal of Attention Disorders, 11*(5), 519–521.

DuPaul, G. J., & Stoner, G. (2014). *ADHD in the schools: Assessment and intervention strategies* (3rd ed.). New York: Guilford Press.

Eiraldi, R., Mazzuca, L., Clarke, A., & Power, T. (2006). Service utilization among ethnic minority children with ADHD: A model of help-seeking behavior. *Administration and Policy in Mental Health and Mental Health Services Research, 33,* 607–622.

Epstein, J. L. (1995). School/family/community partnerships: Caring for the children we share. *Phi Delta Kappan, 76,* 701–712.

Evans, S. W., Langberg, J. M., Schultz, B. K., Vaughn, A., Altaye, M., Marshall, S. A., et al. (2016). Evaluation of a school-based treatment program for young adolescents with ADHD. *Journal of Consulting and Clinical Psychology, 84,* 15–30.

Evans, S. W., Owens, J. S., & Power, T. J. (2019). Attention-deficit/hyperactivity disorder. In M. J. Prinstein, E. A. Youngstrom, E. J. Mash, & R. A. Barkley (Eds.), *Treatment of childhood disorders* (4th ed., pp. 47–101). New York: Guilford Press.

Evans, S. W., Owens, J. S., Wymbs, B. T., & Ray, A. R. (2018). Evidence-based psychosocial treatments for children and adolescents with attention-deficit/hyperactivity disorder. *Journal of Clinical Child and Adolescent Psychology, 47,* 157–198.

Evans, S. W., Schultz, B. K., & DeMars, C. E. (2014). High school-based treatment for adolescents with attention-deficit/hyperactivity disorder: Results from a pilot study examining outcomes and dosage. *School Psychology Review, 43,* 185–202.

Evans, S. W., Schultz, B. K., DeMars, C. E., & Davis, H. (2011). Effectiveness of the challenging horizons after-school program for young adolescents with ADHD. *Behavior Therapy, 42,* 462–474.

Fabiano, G. A., Pelham, W. E., Gnagy, E. M., Burrows-MacLean, L., Chacko, A., Coles, E. K., et al. (2007). The single and combined effects of multiple intensities of behavior modification and multiple intensities of methylphenidate in a classroom setting. *School Psychology Review, 36,* 195–216.

Fabiano, G. A., Pelham, W. E., Waschbusch, D. A., Gnagy, E. M., Lahey, B. B., Chronis, A. M., et al. (2006). A practical measure of impairment: Psychometric properties of the impairment rating scale in samples of children with attention deficit hyperactivity disorder and two school-based samples. *Journal of Clinical Child and Adolescent Psychology, 35,* 369–385.

Fabiano, G. A., Vujnovic, R. K., Pelham, W. E., Waschbusch, D. A., Massetti, G. M., Pariseau, M. E., et al. (2010). Enhancing the effectiveness of special education programming for children with attention deficit hyperactivity disorder using a daily report card. *School Psychology Review, 39,* 219–239.

Fogler, J. M., Normand, S., O'Dea, N., Mautone, J. A., Featherston, M., Power, T. J., et al. (2020). Topical review: Implementing group behavioral parent training in telepsychology: Lessons learned during the COVID-19 pandemic. *Journal of Pediatric Psychology, 45*, 983–989.

Furman, W., & Giberson, R. S. (1995). Identifying the links between parents and their children's sibling relationships. In S. Shuman (Ed.), *Close relationships in social-emotional development* (pp. 95–108). Norwood, NJ: Ablex.

Gormley, M. J., Sheridan, S. M., Dizona, P. J., Witte, A. L., Wheeler, L. A., Eastberg, S. R. A., et al. (2020). Conjoint behavioral consultation for students exhibiting symptoms of ADHD: Effects at post-treatment and one-year follow-up. *School Mental Health, 12*, 53–66.

Hamre, B. K., Pianta, R. C., Downer, J. T., & Mashburn, A. J. (2008). Teachers' perceptions of conflict with young students: Looking beyond problem behaviors. *Social Development, 17*, 115–136.

Harris, P. A., Taylor, R., Thielke, R., Payne, J., Gonzalez, N., & Conde, J. G. (2009). Research electronic data capture (REDCap): A metadata-driven methodology and workflow process for providing translational research informatics support. *Journal of Biomedical Informatics, 42*, 377–381.

Hechtman, L., Swanson, J. M., Sibley M. H., Stehli, A., Owens, E. B., Mitchell, J. T., et al. (2016). Functional adult outcomes 16 years after childhood diagnosis of attention-deficit/hyperactivity disorder: MTA results. *Journal of the American Academy of Child and Adolescent Psychiatry, 55*, 945–952.

Hinshaw, S. P., Owens, E. B., Wells, K. C., Kraemer, H. C., Abikoff, H. B., Arnold, E., et al. (2000). Family processes and treatment outcome in the MTA: Negative/ineffective parent practices in relation to multimodal treatment. *Journal of Abnormal Clinical Child Psychology, 28*, 555–568.

Hook, J. N., Davis, D., Owen, J., & De Blaere, C. (2017). *Cultural humility: Engaging diverse identities in therapy*. Washington, DC: American Psychological Association.

Hoover, S., & Bostic, J. (2021). Schools as a vital component of the child and adolescent mental health system. *Psychiatric Services, 72*, 37–48.

Hoover-Dempsey, K. V., Bassler, O. C., & Brissie, J. S. (1992). Explorations in parent–school relations. *Journal of Educational Research, 85*, 287–294.

Ingoldsby, E. M. (2010). Review of interventions to improve family engagement and retention in parent and child mental health programs. *Journal of Child and Family Studies, 19*, 629–645.

Johnston, C., Mash, E. J., Miller, N., & Ninowski, J. E. (2012). Parenting in adults with attention deficit/hyperactivity disorder (ADHD). *Clinical Psychology Review, 32*, 215–228.

Kazantzis, N., Whittington, C., & Dattilio, F. (2010). Meta-analysis of homework effects in cognitive and behavioral therapy: A replication and extension. *Clinical Psychology: Science and Practice, 17*, 144–156.

Kazdin, A. E. (2005). *Parent management training: Treatment for oppositional, aggressive, and antisocial behavior in children and adolescents*. New York: Oxford University Press.

Kohl, G. O., Lengua, L. J., McMahon, R. J., & Conduct Problems Prevention Research Group. (2000). Parent involvement in school: Conceptualizing multiple dimensions and their relations with family and demographic risk factors. *Journal of School Psychology, 38*, 501–523.

Kolko, D. J., Campo, J., Kilbourne, A. M., Hart, J., Sakolsky, D., & Wisniewski, S. (2014). Collaborative care outcomes for pediatric behavioral health problems: A cluster randomized trial. *Pediatrics, 133*(4), e981–e992.

Koshy, A. J., Mautone, J. A., Pendergast, L. L., Blum, N. J., & Power, T. J. (2016). Validation of the Behavioral Health Checklist in urban and suburban pediatric primary care setting. *Journal of Developmental and Behavioral Pediatrics, 37*, 132–139.

Kotowski, S. E., Davis, K. G., & Barratt, C. L. (2022). Teachers feeling the burden of COVID-19: Impact on well-being, stress, and burnout. *Work, 71*, 407–415.

Krain, A. L., Kendall, P. C., & Power, T. J. (2005). The role of treatment acceptability in the initiation of treatment for ADHD. *Journal of Attention Disorders, 9*, 425–434.

Langberg, J. M., Arnold, L. E., Flowers, A. M., Epstein, J. N., Altaye, M., Hinshaw, S. P., et al. (2010). Parent-reported homework problems in the MTA study: Evidence for sustained improvement with behavioral treatment. *Journal of Clinical Child and Adolescent Psychology, 39*, 220–233.

Langberg, J. M., Dvorsky, M. R., Molitor, S. J., Bourchtein, E., Eddy, L. D., Smith, Z. R., et al. (2018). Overcoming the research-to-practice gap: A randomized trial with two brief homework and organization interventions for students with ADHD as implemented by school mental health providers. *Journal of Consulting and Clinical Psychology, 86*, 39–55.

Langberg, J. M., Epstein, J. N., Becker, S. P., Girio-Herrera, E., & Vaughn, A. J. (2012). Evaluation of the homework, organization, and planning skills (HOPS) intervention for middle school students with attention deficits hyperactivity disorder as implemented by school mental health providers. *School Psychology Review, 41*, 342–364.

Langberg, J. M., Molina, B. S. G., Arnold, L. E., Epstein, J. N., Altaye, M., Hinshaw, S., et al. (2011). Patterns and predictors of adolescent academic achievement and performance in a sample of children with attention-deficit/hyperactivity disorder. *Journal of Clinical Child and Adolescent Psychology, 40*(4), 1–13.

Mautone, J. A., Marcelle, E., Tresco, K. E., & Power, T. J. (2015). Assessing the quality of parent–teacher relationships for students with ADHD. *Psychology in the Schools, 52*(2), 196–207.

Mautone, J. A., Marshall, S. A., Sharman, J., Eiraldi, R. B., Jawad, A. F., & Power, T. J. (2012). Development of a family-school intervention for young children with ADHD. *School Psychology Review, 41*, 447–466.

Mautone, J. A., Pendergast, L. L., Cassano, M., Blum, N. J., & Power, T. J. (2020). Behavioral health screening: Validation of a strength-based approach. *Journal of Developmental and Behavioral Pediatrics, 41*, 587–595.

McMahon, R. J., & Forehand, R. L. (2003). *Helping the noncompliant child: Family-based treatment for oppositional behavior* (2nd ed.). New York: Guilford Press.

Merrill, B. M., Morrow, A. S., Altszuler, A. R., Macphee, F. L., Gnagy, E. M., Greiner, A. R., et al. (2017). Improving homework performance among children with ADHD: A randomized clinical trial. *Journal of Consulting and Clinical Psychology, 85*, 111–122.

Miller, S., & Rollnick, W. R. (2023). *Motivational interviewing: Helping people change and grow* (4th ed.). New York: Guilford Press.

Morris, S., Nahmias, A., Nissley-Tsiopinis, J., Orapallo, A., Power, T. J., & Mautone, J. A. (2019). Research to practice: Implementation of Family–School Success for parents of children with ADHD. *Cognitive and Behavioral Practice, 24*, 983–989.

MTA Cooperative Group. (1999). Moderators and mediators of treatment response for children with attention-deficit/hyperactivity disorder. *Archives of General Psychiatry, 56*, 1088–1096.

Nissley-Tsiopinis, J., Normand, S., Mautone, J. A., Fogler, J. M., Featherston, M., & Power, T. J. (2023). Preparing families for evidence-based treatment of ADHD: Development of bootcamp for ADHD. *Cognitive and Behavioral Practice, 30*(3), 453–470.

Nissley-Tsiopinis, J., Tresco, K. E., Mautone, J. A., & Power, T. J. (2014, November). *Moderators and predictors of combined family-school intervention for children with ADHD: The influence of child and family characteristics*. Presented at annual meeting of the Association for Behavior and Cognitive Therapies, Philadelphia, PA.

Nix, R. L., Bierman, K. L., & McMahon, R. J. (2009). How attendance and quality of participation affect treatment response to parent management training. *Journal of Consulting and Clinical Psychology, 77*, 429–438.

Nixon, S. A. (2019). The coin model of privilege and critical allyship: Implications for health. *BMC Public Health, 19*, 1637.

Owens, J. S., Holdaway, A. S., Zoromski, A. K., Evans, S. W., Himawan, L. K., Girio-Herrera, E., et al. (2012). Incremental benefits of a daily report card intervention over time for youth with disruptive behavior. *Behavior Therapy, 43*, 848–861.

Patterson GR. (1982). *Coercive family process*. Eugene, OR: Castalia.

Pelham, W. E., Jr., & Fabiano, G. A. (2008). Evidence-based psychosocial treatments for attention-deficit/hyperactivity disorder. *Journal of Clinical Child and Adolescent Psychology, 37*, 184–214.

Pelham, W. E., Jr., Fabiano, G. A., Waxmonsky, J. G., Greiner, A. R., Gnagy, E. M., Pelham, W. E., III, et al. (2016). Treatment sequencing for childhood ADHD: A multiple-randomization study of adaptive medication and behavioral interventions. *Journal of Clinical Child and Adolescent Psychology, 45*, 396–415.

Pelham, W. E., Jr., Wheeler, T., & Chronis, A. (1998). Empirically supported psychosocial treatments for attention deficit hyperactivity disorder. *Journal of Clinical Child Psychology, 27*, 190–205.

Pennotti, R., Lawson, G., Mautone, J. A., Rosenquist, R., Rubin, D., & Young, J. F. (2022). *Building and sustaining programs for school-based behavioral health services in K–12 schools*. PolicyLab, Children's Hospital of Philadelphia, Philadelphia, PA. Retrieved from *https://policylab.chop.edu/sites/default/files/pdf/publications/PolicyLab-Paper-Building-Sustaining-Programs-School-based-BH-Services-K12-Schools.pdf*.

Pfiffner, L. J., Hinshaw, S. P., Owens, E., Zalecki, C., Kaiser, N. M., Villodas, M., et al. (2014). A two-site randomized clinical trial of integrated psychosocial treatment for ADHD-inattentive type. *Journal of Consulting and Clinical Psychology, 82*, 1115–1127.

Pfiffner, L. J., Rooney, M. E., Jiang, Y., Haack, L. M., Beaulieu, A., & McBurnett, K. (2018). Sustained effects of collaborative school-home intervention for attention-deficit/hyperactivity disorder symptoms and impairment. *Journal of the American Academy of Child and Adolescent Psychiatry, 57*, 245–251.

Pfiffner, L. J., Villodas, M., Kaiser, N., Rooney, M., & McBurnett, K. (2013). Educational outcomes of a collaborative school–home behavioral intervention in ADHD. *School Psychology Quarterly, 28*, 25–36.

Pianta, R. C. (1999). *Enhancing relationships between children and teachers*. Washington, DC: American Psychological Association.

Power, T., Blom-Hoffman, J., Clarke, A., Riley-Tillman, C., Kelleher, C., & Manz, P. (2005). Reconceptualizing intervention integrity: A partnership-based framework for linking research with practice. *Psychology in the Schools, 42*, 495–507.

Power, T. J., Blum, N. J., Guevara, J. P., Jones, H. A., & Leslie, L. K. (2013). Coordinating mental health care across primary care and schools: ADHD as a case example. *Advances in School Mental Health Promotion, 6,* 68–80.

Power, T. J., & Bradley-Klug, K. (2013). *Pediatric school psychology: Conceptualization, applications, and strategies for leadership development.* New York: Routledge.

Power, T. J., Karustis, J. L., & Habboushe, D. (2001). *Homework success for children with ADHD: A family–school intervention program.* New York: Guilford Press.

Power, T. J., Koshy, A. J., Watkins, M. W., Cassano, M. C., Wahlberg, A. C., Mautone, J. A., et al. (2013). Developmentally and culturally appropriate screening in primary care: Development of the Behavioral Health Checklist. *Journal of Pediatric Psychology, 38,* 1155–1164.

Power, T. J., Mautone, J. A., Marshall, S. A., Jones, H. A., Cacia, J., Tresco, K. E., et al. (2014). Feasibility and potential effectiveness of integrated services for children with ADHD in urban primary care practices. *Clinical Practice in Pediatric Psychology, 2,* 412–426.

Power, T. J., Mautone, J. A., Soffer, S. L., Clarke, A. T., Marshall, S. A., Sharman, J., et al. (2012). Family-school intervention for children with ADHD: Results of randomized clinical trial. *Journal of Consulting and Clinical Psychology, 80,* 611–623.

Power, T. J., Watkins, M. W., Anastopoulos, A. D., Reid, R., Lambert, M. C., & DuPaul, G. J. (2017). Multi-informant assessment of ADHD symptom-related impairments among children and adolescents. *Journal of Clinical Child and Adolescent Psychology, 46,* 661–674.

Power, T. J., Watkins, M. W., Mautone, J. A., Walcott, C. M., Coutts, M. J., & Sheridan, S. M. (2015). Examining the validity of the Homework Performance Questionnaire: Multi-informant assessment in elementary and middle school. *School Psychology Quarterly, 30,* 260–275.

Power, T., Werba, B., Watkins, M., Angelucci, J., & Eiraldi, R. (2006). Patterns of parent-reported homework problems among ADHD-referred and nonreferred children. *School Psychology Quarterly, 21,* 13–33.

Rooney, M., Hinshaw, S. McBurnett, K., & Pfiffner, L. J. (2018). Parent adherence in two behavioral treatment strategies for the predominantly inattentive presentation of ADHD. *Journal of Clinical Child and Adolescent Psychology, 47,* S233–S241.

Ryan, R. M., & Deci, E. L. (2008). A self-determination theory approach to psychotherapy: The motivational basis for effective change. *Canadian Psychology, 49,* 186–193.

Ryan, R. M., & Deci, E. L. (2018). *Self-determination theory: Basic psychological needs in motivation, development, and wellness.* New York: Guilford Press.

Shahidullah, J. D., Hostutler, C. A., Coker, T. R., Allmon Dixson, A., Okoroji, C., & Mautone, J. A. (2023). Child health equity and primary care. *American Psychologist, 78,* 93–106.

Shahidullah, J. D., Hostutler, C. A., & Stancin, T. (2018). Collaborative medication-related roles for pediatric primary care psychologists. *Clinical Practice in Pediatric Psychology, 6,* 61–72.

Sheridan, S. M., Bovaird, J. A., Glover, T. A., Garbacz, S. A., Witte, A., & Kwon, K. (2012). A randomized trial examining the effects of conjoint behavioral consultation and the mediating role of the parent–teacher relationship, *School Psychology Review, 41,* 23–46,

Sheridan, S. M., Clarke, B. L., & Ransom, K. A. (2014). The past, present, and future of conjoint behavioral consultation research. In W. P. Erchul & S. M. Sheridan (Eds.), *Handbook of research in school consultation* (pp. 210–247). New York: Routledge/Taylor & Francis Group.

Sheridan, S. M., & Kratochwill. T. R. (2007). *Conjoint behavioral consultation: Promoting family–school connections and interventions* (2nd ed.). New York: Springer.

Sheridan, S. M., Witte, A. L., Holmes, S. R., Coutts, M. J., Dent, A. L., Kunza, G. M., et al. (2017). A randomized trial examining the effects of conjoint behavioral consultation in rural schools: Student outcomes and the mediating role of the teacher–parent relationship. *Journal of School Psychology, 61,* 33–53.

Sibley, M. H. (2016). *Parent–teen therapy for executive function deficits and ADHD: Building skills and motivation.* New York: Guilford Press.

Sibley, M. H., Graziano, P. A., Kuriyan, A. B., Coxe, S., Pelham, W. E., Rodriguez, L., et al. (2016). Parent–teen behavior therapy + motivational interviewing for adolescents with ADHD. *Journal of Consulting and Clinical Psychology, 84,* 699–712.

Skinner, B. F. (1976). *About behaviorism.* New York: Random House.

Smith, J. D., Cruden, G. H., Rojas, L. M., Van Ryzin, M., Fu, E., Davis, M. M., et al. (2020). Parenting interventions in pediatric primary care: A systematic review. *Pediatrics, 146,* e20193548.

Sonuga-Barke E. J., Daley D., & Thompson M. (2002). Does maternal ADHD reduce the effectiveness of parent training for preschool children's ADHD? *Journal of the American Academy of Child and Adolescent Psychiatry, 41,* 696–702.

Sonuga-Barke, E. J. S., Daley, D., Thompson, M., Laver-Bradbury, C., & Weeks, A. (2001). Parent-based therapies for preschool attention-deficit/hyperactivity disorder: A randomized, controlled trial with a community sample. *Journal of the American Academy of Child and Adolescent Psychiatry, 40,* 402–408.

Sroufe, L. A. (2016). The place of attachment in development. In J. Cassidy & P. R. Shaver (Eds.), *Handbook of attachment: Theory, research, and clinical applications* (3rd ed., pp. 997–1011). New York: Guilford Press.

Sroufe, L. A., Carlson, E. A., Levy, A. K., & Egeland, B. (1999). Implications of attachment theory for developmental psychopathology. *Development and Psychopathology, 11*, 1–13.

Sroufe, L. A., Egeland, B., Carlson, E. A., & Collins, W. A. (2005). *The development of the person: The Minnesota Study of Risk and Adaptation from Birth to Adulthood.* New York: Guilford Press.

Takeda, T., Stotebery, K., Power, T. J., Ambrosini, P., Beretini, W., Hakonarson, H., et al. (2010). Parental ADHD status and its association with proband, ADHD subtype and severity. *Journal of Pediatrics, 157*, 995–1000.

Visser, S. N., Danielson, M. L., Bitsko, R. H., Holbrook, J. R., Kogan, M. D., Ghandour, R. M., et al. (2014). Trends in the parent-report of health care provider-diagnosed and medicated attention-deficit/hyperactivity disorder: United States, 2003–2011. *Journal of the American Academy of Child and Adolescent Psychiatry, 53*(1), 34–46.

Volpe, R. J., & Fabiano, G. A. (2013). *Daily behavior report cards: An evidence-based system of assessment and intervention.* New York: Guilford Press.

Webster-Stratton, C., & Hammond, M. (1997). Treating children with early-onset conduct problems: A comparison of child and parent interventions. *Journal of Consulting and Clinical Psychology, 65*, 93–109.

Weisenmuller, C., & Hilton, D. (2020). Barriers to access, implementation, and utilization of parenting interventions: Considerations for research and clinical applications. *American Psychologist, 76*, 104–115.

Wells, K. C., Epstein, J. N., Hinshaw, S. P., Conners, C. K., Klaric, J., Abikoff, H. B., et al. (2000). Parenting and family stress treatment outcomes in attention deficit hyperactivity disorder (ADHD): An empirical analysis in the MTA study. *Journal of Abnormal Child Psychology, 28*, 543–553.

Wolraich, M. L., Hagan, J. F., Jr., Allan, C., Chan, E., Davison, D., Earls, M., et al. (2019). Clinical practice guideline for the diagnosis, evaluation, and treatment of attention-deficit/hyperactivity disorder in children and adolescents. *Pediatrics, 144*(4), e20192528.

Index

Note. *f* or *t* following a page number indicates a figure or a table.

A-B-C analysis. *See also* A-B-C's of behavior
    challenging situations and, 116–117
    homework problems and, 90–91, 97
    overview, 64
    between-session practice with, 68
A-B-C's of behavior. *See also* A-B-C analysis
    challenging situations and, 116–117
    helping parents understand, 63–64
    homework problems and, 90–91, 97
    overview, 171
    reviewing homework on, 71–72
    between-session practice with, 67–68
Academic performance, 27*t*, 28, 48
Academic Proficiency Scale (APS), 140, 242
Acceptability of FSS, 20–21, 25
Adaptations to FSS
    delivering in primary care practices, 9, 126
    individualized family sessions, 29–30, 128–129
    offering FSS in the summer, 130
    offering in private practice, 126–127
    for older or younger students, 26, 129–130
    overview, 9, 125, 131
    telehealth methods and, 9, 31, 127–128
    varying family constellations, 130–131
Adherence, 137
Adolescents, 129–130
Age of child, 26, 27*t*, 129–130
Antecedent strategy. *See also* Antecedents of behavior
    challenging situations and, 116–117
    establishing a homework ritual, 91–92
    overview, 64–65
    reviewing homework on, 71–72
Antecedents of behavior, 63–64, 71–72, 90–91. *See also* Antecedent strategy

Anxiety and anxiety disorders, 23, 27, 48
Appropriateness of FSS, 26–27, 27*t*
Assessment of child safety, 34
Attachment theory, 6, 13–14
Attendance, 24, 137
Attending, strategic, 49. *See also* Attention when parenting
Attention when parenting
    homework regarding, 50, 54
    overview, 49, 164
    as reinforcement, 81
Attention-deficit/hyperactivity disorder (ADHD)
    appropriateness of FSS and, 26–27, 27*t*
    overview, 3–4, 160–163
    reviewing with parents, 48
Autism spectrum disorder (ASD), 27, 27*t*, 48
Autonomous motivation, 14–15
Aversive consequences. *See* Consequences of behavior; Punishment

Barriers to care, 38, 54
Behavior change, 109
Behavior management, 65–66, 208–209
Behavioral consultation. *See* Conjoint behavioral consultation (CBC)
Behavioral contingency management. *See* Classroom behavioral intervention
Behavioral functioning
    appropriateness of FSS and, 27*t*
    challenging situations and, 116–117
    Child's Game and, 58
    effects of ADHD on, 48
Behavioral health care, 9
Behavioral Health Checklist (BHCL), 138–139, 144, 148–149, 233–234

Behavioral homework interventions. *See* Homework performance
Behavioral parent training (BPT)
　empirical support for, 6, 11
　overview, 4–5, 4t, 15, 16, 17t
　treatment response and, 23
Behavioral psychology, 5–6, 12–13
Between-session homework for parents. *See also individual sessions*
　A-B-C analysis, 67–68, 71–72, 92–93, 97
　challenges during FSS sessions and strategies to provide support, 40t
　Child's Game, 58, 62–63, 67–68, 71–72, 81, 90, 98, 102, 107, 111, 116
　Coding Manual for FSS Between-Session Homework Assignments, 245–248
　completion of, 137
　daily report card (DRC), 76–77, 81
　goal-setting strategy, 102, 106, 111, 115
　home–school collaboration, 76–77, 80–81, 102, 106–107
　homework problems, 92–93, 97–98, 102, 106–107, 115
　overview, 7
　parental engagement and, 24, 25, 137
　parental implementation of strategies and, 8
　positive attending, 50, 54
　punishment, 110–111, 115
　strategies to promote family engagement and, 37–38
　support from others, 71–72
　token economies, 85, 89–90, 97–98
"Big Ideas," 47, 158
Bribery, 66

Caregivers, support from. *See* Support of other caregivers
Catch them being good technique, 49, 165–166
Challenging situations, 116–117, 201
Change talk, 135–136
Child abuse, 34
Child group sessions. *See also* Group delivery; *individual sessions*
　overview, 44
　session 1 (intro to the FSS program), 50–51
　session 2 (strengthening family relationships), 59–60
　session 3 (basics of behavior management), 68–69
　session 4 (preparing for family–school collaboration), 77–78
　session 5 (introducing the token economy), 85–87
　session 6 (function of behavior and establishing the homework ritual), 93–95
　session 7 (managing time and goal setting), 102–104
　session 9 (planning for future success), 119–121
　telehealth methods and, 128
Child outcomes, 133t. *See also* Evaluating outcomes
Children
　adapting FSS for use with younger or older students, 129–130
　appropriateness of FSS and, 26–27, 27t
　involving in FSS, 8–9, 30, 44
　measures of child outcomes, 138–140
　protecting family privacy and safety and, 34
　skills training and, 16–17
　telehealth methods and, 128

Child's Game, 56–58, 60, 62–63, 168–169. *See also* Between-session homework for parents; *individual sessions*
Classroom behavioral intervention
　empirical support for, 6, 11
　homework problems and, 17
　overview, 4t, 5, 17–18, 17t
Classroom-focused intervention strategies, 28
Coding Manual for FSS Between-Session Homework Assignments, 245–248
Coexisting conditions, 27, 27t, 48
Cognitive processing, 18–19
Cognitive behavioral therapy, 27
Cognitive behavioral training approaches, 19
Collaboration between families and schools. *See* Family–school relationships; Home–school collaboration; Session 4 (preparing for family–school collaboration)
Commands. *See* Directions, giving to children
Communication, 64–65, 73–74, 75–76
Completion of FSS, 119, 120–121
Concentration Game, 94, 112–113
Conduct disorder, 27, 27t
Conducting sessions. *See* Sessions
Confidentiality, 34
Conjoint behavioral consultation (CBC), 4t, 5, 6, 17, 17t, 28
Consent, 35, 47–48
Consequence strategies, 65–66, 116–117. *See also* Consequences of behavior; Positive reinforcement; Reinforcement
Consequences of behavior. *See also* Consequence strategies; Punishment
　child group sessions and, 69
　discussing with children, 112–113
　helping parents understand, 63–64
　homework problems and, 90–91
　overview, 173–174
　reviewing homework regarding, 71–72, 115–116
Content fidelity, 41, 134. *See also* Fidelity
Contextual influences, 14, 28
Contingency management, 11. *See also* Classroom behavioral intervention
Coping and organizational strategies for parents, 4t, 5, 17t, 18–19, 40t, 55–56
Coping with ADHD through Relationships and Education (CARE), 19–20
Cultural humility, 10, 38–39

Daily report card (DRC). *See also* Classroom behavioral intervention
　guidelines for establishing, 75–76, 182
　homework problems and, 17
　overview, 17t, 18
　reviewing homework on, 80–81
　between-session practice with, 76–77, 80–81
Debriefing after sessions, 39, 41
Depression, 27, 40t
Didactic presentation, 36
Directions, giving to children, 57, 64–65, 172

Discipline strategies, 11. *See also* Punishment
Discussion, group. *See* Group discussion
Diversity, 38–39
Dysregulation, 117

Early education, 9, 129
Ecological systems theory, 6, 14
Educational performance. *See* Academic performance
Effectiveness of FSS, 21, 22*f*, 23*f*, 25
Emotional control, 110, 117
Emotional validation, 136
Empowerment, 35, 36, 41
Engagement
  Child's Game and, 58
  family engagement, 137
  measures of, 133*t*, 137
  parental engagement and, 24, 25
  process fidelity and, 135
  promoting parent self-discovery and empowerment and, 35
  strategies to promote, 37–38
  telehealth methods and, 128
Environmental factors, 13, 47, 49
Evaluating outcomes. *See also* Fidelity; Intervention evaluation
  measures for, 137–140, 231–248
  overview, 132–134, 133*t*, 140–141, 142, 144, 146*t*, 147–151
Evidence-based interventions, 3–4, 11–12, 48
Example of FSS implementation
  context of, 143
  outcome results, 144–145, 146*t*
  overview, 142, 147–151
  participants and intervention procedures, 143–144
Executive-functioning training approaches, 19
Extinction burst, 12–13, 49

Fabulous Four Game, 94–95
Family behavioral interventions, 23
Family engagement, 37–38, 137, 145, 146*t*. *See also* Engagement
Family involvement in education, 15, 16*f*, 17*t*, 48–49
Family relationships, 4, 11. *See also* Parent–child relationships; Relationship functioning
Family sessions, individualized, 29–30, 128–129
Family–school relationships. *See also* Home–school collaboration; Relationship functioning; Session 4 (preparing for family–school collaboration)
  appropriateness of FSS and, 28
  homework problems and, 16
  implementation of FSS in schools and, 28
  measures of outcomes and, 137–138
  overview, 4, 24–25
  permissions to communicate with teachers and, 35, 47–48
  between-session practice with, 76–77
Family–School Success (FSS) program overview. *See also* Child group sessions; *individual sessions*
  children and families appropriate for, 26–27, 27*t*
  completion of, 119

  components of, 4–5
  empirical support for, 6, 15–19, 15*f*, 16*t*
  examples of implementation and outcomes, 142–151, 146*t*
  implementation in schools, 28
  including children in, 8–9, 30
  introducing to parents, 46–48
  overview, 3, 11–12, 24–25, 29–30, 32
  process fidelity and, 136
  recruiting families for, 29
  research on, 19–25, 22*f*, 23*f*
  theoretical justifications for, 5–6, 12–15
  who can provide, 31–32
Family–School Success Program Evaluation Scale, 140, 144–145, 243–244
Feasibility of FSS, 20–21, 25, 28
Fidelity. *See also* Evaluating outcomes
  checklists for, 7, 219–228
  debriefing following sessions and, 39, 41
  implementation of FSS and, 36–37, 41
  measures of, 133*t*, 134–137, 135*t*
Financial factors to implementation, 28, 29, 31
Flexibility, 36–37
Formula for Success, 118, 120, 203–205

Genetic factors, 48
Goal setting. *See also* Session 7 (managing time and goal setting)
  child group sessions and, 103–104
  developing using modeling, role play, and guided practice, 99–101
  overview, 14–15, 195–196
  reviewing homework on practice of, 106–107, 112, 115–116
Group delivery. *See also* Child group sessions; *individual sessions*
  balancing didactic presentation and group discussion in, 36
  factors to consider in organizing groups, 31
  format of, 43–44
  overview, 29–30
  protecting family privacy and safety during, 34
  time management during, 34
Group discussion, 36, 40*t*
Guided practice, 99–101

Handouts for parents
  overview, 7
  for session 1, 45, 155–167
  for session 2, 53, 168–170
  for session 3, 61–62, 171–180
  for session 4, 70, 181–185
  for session 5, 79, 186–190
  for session 6, 88, 186–194
  for session 7, 96, 195–197
  for session 8, 105, 198–200
  for session 9, 114, 201–215
Harm to others, 34
Healthcare settings, 9, 28, 29, 126–127
Home environment, 13, 47, 49

Home–school collaboration. *See also* Family–school relationships; Schools; Session 4 (preparing for family–school collaboration); Teachers
  establishing a daily report card (DRC) and, 75–76
  homework problems and, 92, 99, 102
  importance of, 72–73
  overview, 24–25, 47
  partnerships with teachers and, 73–74, 181
  between-session practice with, 76–77, 80–81, 106–107
Homework between sessions. *See* Between-session homework for parents
Homework performance. *See also* Session 6 (function of behavior and establishing the homework ritual)
  antecedents and consequences of homework behavior, 90–91
  appropriateness of FSS and, 27*t*
  behavioral homework interventions, 4*t*, 5, 6, 16–17, 17*t*
  child group sessions and, 94, 103–104
  homework rituals and, 91–92, 191–192
  modifying FSS for use with families of young children, 129
  between-session practice regarding, 97–98, 115–116
  time limits for doing homework, 98–99
  time management and goal-setting skills and, 99–101, 102
Homework Performance Questionnaire—Parent Version (HPQ-P), 139, 144, 150, 235–238
Homework Performance Questionnaire—Teacher Version (HPQ-T), 139, 239–241
Homework Problem Checklist (HPC), 139

Ignoring
  behavioral psychology theory and, 12–13
  Child's Game and, 58
  compared to punishment, 66, 108
  with dysregulated children, 117
  impact of, 49
  overview, 174
Imitation, 13, 57
Impairment Rating Scale—Parent Version (IRS-P), 139, 144, 149–150
Impairment Rating Scale—Teacher Version (IRS-T), 140
Implementation of FSS. *See also* Example of FSS implementation; Fidelity
  appropriateness of FSS and, 26–27, 27*t*
  factors to consider in organizing groups, 31
  with fidelity and flexibility, 36–37
  in groups or individually, 29–30
  in health and mental health settings, 28
  overview, 32, 42
  promoting parent self-discovery and empowerment and, 35
  in schools, 28
  who can provide FSS, 31–32
  working with families from diverse backgrounds, 38–39
Individual delivery of interventions, 29–30, 128–129
Instructions, giving to children, 57, 64–65, 172
Internalizing symptoms, 27, 27*t*
Intervention evaluation. *See also* Evaluating outcomes; Fidelity
  conjoint behavioral consultation and, 17
  example of FSS implementation and, 145–151, 146*t*
  overview, 132–134, 133*t*

Kindergarten-age children, 129

Learning and learning disabilities, 13, 48
Listening, 18, 64–65

Managing time. *See* Session 7 (managing time and goal setting); Time management skills
Medication. *See* Pharmacological interventions
Mental health settings, 9, 28, 29, 31–32
Modeling, 13, 74, 99–101
Motivation, 14–15, 128
Motivational interviewing (MI)
  empirical support for, 6
  overview, 4, 4*t*, 5, 17*t*, 18
  parental engagement and, 24
  self-determination theory and, 14–15
  time management and goal-setting skills and, 101
Multimodal Treatment of ADHD study, 23

Negative punishment, 12–13, 108–109. *See also* Punishment
Negative reinforcement, 12, 65–66. *See also* Punishment; Reinforcement
Neurobiology of ADHD, 48

Observing others, 13
Older students, 129–130
Online delivery. *See* Telehealth methods
Oppositional defiant disorder, 27, 27*t*, 48
Organizational skills of parents. *See* Coping and organizational strategies for parents; Parental coping and organization
Organizational skills training, 11, 18–19
Outcomes. *See* Evaluating outcomes

Parent as Educator Scale (PES), 138
Parent training, 16–17. *See also* Coping and organizational strategies for parents
Parental ADHD, 4, 9. *See also* Family relationships
Parental coping and organization. *See* Coping and organizational strategies for parents
Parental engagement in FSS, 24, 137
Parental implementation of strategies, 8
Parent–Child Questionnaire, 231–232
Parent–Child Relationship Questionnaire (PCRQ), 137–138, 144, 147–148
Parent–child relationships
  appropriateness of FSS and, 27*t*
  attachment theory and, 13
  "Big Ideas" and, 47
  Child's Game and, 56–57
  homework problems and, 16
  overview, 4
  play and, 56–57
  strengthening, 15, 16*f*, 17*t*
Parenting practices
  attachment theory and, 13
  behavioral parent training and, 11
  overview, 55–56
  parent effectiveness, 15, 16*f*, 17*t*
  strengthening, 15, 16*f*, 17*t*

Parents, 35, 47–48
Parent–teacher collaboration. *See* Home–school collaboration
Parent–Teacher Involvement Questionnaire (PTIQ), 138, 144, 148
Peer relationships, 27t
Pharmacological interventions, 3–4, 11
Planning skills training, 11, 18–19
Play, 56–57. *See also* Child's Game
Positive attending. *See* Attention when parenting; Session 1 (intro to the FSS program)
Positive punishment, 12–13, 109. *See also* Punishment
Positive reinforcement. *See also* Reinforcement; Token economies
   behavioral psychology theory and, 12
   child group sessions and, 52
   consequence strategies and, 65–66
   overview, 81, 175–178
   removal of in punishment, 108–109
   reviewing homework on, 71–72
   types of reinforcers, 67, 81
Praise, 57, 81
Preschool-age children, 9, 129
PRIDE skills, 57
Primary care practices, 9, 126. *See also* Healthcare settings
Private practice, 126–127
Pro Tips, 43–44
Problem identification and analysis, 17
Process fidelity, 41, 134–136, 135t, 228. *See also* Fidelity
Program satisfaction, 133t, 144–145
Proximal outcomes, 133t. *See also* Evaluating outcomes
Psychosocial interventions, 3–4, 11
Public places, behavior in, 117
Punishment. *See also* Consequences of behavior; Negative reinforcement; Reinforcement; Session 8 (using punishment successfully)
   A-B-C's of behavior and, 64
   behavioral psychology theory and, 12–13
   child group sessions and, 69
   compared to ignoring, 66, 108
   discussing with children, 112–113
   with dysregulated children, 117
   homework regarding, 110–111
   implementing successfully, 108–110, 198
   introducing to parents, 107–108
   overview, 173–174
   reviewing homework regarding, 115–116
   social learning theory and, 13

Rating systems for daily report cards, 75. *See also* Daily report card (DRC)
Recruitment strategies, 29, 126–127
Reinforcement. *See also* Positive reinforcement; Punishment; Token economies
   A-B-C's of behavior and, 64
   behavioral psychology theory and, 12
   overview, 173
   between-session practice with, 67–68, 71–72
   social learning theory and, 13
   types of reinforcers, 67, 81

Relationship functioning, 4, 27t. *See also* Parent–child relationships; Teacher–student relationships
Resistance, 18, 101
Reward Guessing Game, 86–87
Rewards. *See also* Classroom behavioral intervention; Reinforcement; Token economies
   behavioral psychology theory and, 12
   child group sessions and, 69
   identifying, 82–83, 87
Role playing
   child group sessions and, 87, 104
   Child's Game and, 57–58
   partnerships with teachers and, 74
   time management and goal-setting skills and, 99–101, 104, 112
Rolling with resistance, 18, 101

Safety, 34, 47
Scheduling factors, 28, 29, 31
Schools. *See also* Home–school collaboration
   implementation of FSS in, 28
   permissions to communicate with, 35, 47–48
   recruitment strategies and, 29
Self-determination theory (SDT), 6, 14–15, 35
Self-discovery, parent, 35, 36, 41
Self-empowerment. *See* Empowerment
Self-harm, 34
Session 1 (intro to the FSS program)
   agenda for, 45, 50
   child group, 50–52
   fidelity checklist for, 219
   goals for, 46–52
   materials and handouts for, 45–46, 50, 155–167
   process reminders, 46
Session 2 (strengthening family relationships)
   agenda for, 53, 59
   child group, 59–60
   fidelity checklist for, 220
   goals for, 54–58, 59–60
   materials and handouts for, 53, 59, 168–170
   process reminders, 54
Session 3 (basics of behavior management)
   agenda for, 61, 68
   child group, 68–69
   fidelity checklist for, 221
   goals for, 62–69
   materials and handouts for, 61–62, 68, 171–180
   process reminders, 62
   for session 3, 61–62
Session 4 (preparing for family–school collaboration)
   agenda for, 70, 77
   child group, 77–78
   fidelity checklist for, 222
   goals for, 71–78
   materials and handouts for, 70, 77, 181–185
   process reminders, 71
Session 5 (introducing the token economy)
   agenda for, 79, 85
   child group, 85–87
   fidelity checklist for, 223
   goals for, 80–87

Session 5 (introducing the token economy) *(cont.)*
  materials and handouts for, 79, 85, 186–190
  process reminders, 80
Session 6 (function of behavior and establishing the homework ritual)
  agenda for, 88, 93
  child group, 93–95
  fidelity checklist for, 224
  goals for, 89–95
  materials and handouts for, 88, 186–194
  materials for, 93
  process reminders, 89
Session 7 (managing time and goal setting)
  agenda for, 96, 102
  child group, 102–104
  fidelity checklist for, 225
  goals for, 97–102, 103–104
  materials and handouts for, 96, 102–103, 195–197
  process reminders, 97
Session 8 (using punishment successfully)
  agenda for, 105, 111
  child group, 111–113
  fidelity checklist for, 226
  goals for, 106–113
  materials and handouts for, 105, 111, 198–200
  process reminders, 105–106
Session 9 (planning for future success)
  agenda for, 114, 119
  child group, 119–121
  fidelity checklist for, 227
  goals for, 115–119, 120–121
  materials and handouts for, 114, 119, 201–215
  process reminders, 115
Session-by-session manual, 7, 33, 41–42, 43–44. *See also* Sessions; *individual sessions*
Sessions. *See also individual sessions*
  balancing didactic presentation and group discussion in, 36
  debriefing following, 39, 41
  family engagement and, 37–38
  format of, 43–44
  parent self-discovery and empowerment and, 35
  parents who experience challenges during, 39, 40*t*–41*t*
  permissions to communicate with teachers, 35
  preparation for, 33
  protecting family privacy and safety during, 34
  time management during, 34
  working with families from diverse backgrounds, 38–39
Skepticism, 40*t*, 101
Skills training, 4, 11, 17
Social functioning, 48
Social learning theory, 6, 13

Strategic attending, 49. *See also* Attention when parenting
Strategic ignoring, 49. *See also* Ignoring
Stress, 14, 24, 40*t*, 55
Summer programs, 130
Supervision, 32
Support of other caregivers, 55–56, 72, 136
Supporting self-efficacy, 18

Target behaviors
  A-B-C's of behavior and, 63–64
  consequence strategies and, 65–66
  developing a token economy and, 83
  establishing a daily report card (DRC) and, 75–76
Teacher–home collaboration. *See* Home–school collaboration
Teachers. *See also* Home–school collaboration; Teacher–student relationships
  partnerships with, 73–74, 181
  permissions to communicate with, 35, 47–48
Teacher–student relationships. *See also* Teachers
  appropriateness of FSS and, 27*t*
  attachment theory and, 14
  importance of, 72–73, 78
  overview, 4
Telehealth methods, 9, 31, 127–128. *See also* Example of FSS implementation
Theory, 5–6, 12–15
Theory of change, 47, 54, 159
Time management during FSS sessions, 34
Time management skills. *See also* Session 7 (managing time and goal setting)
  developing using modeling, role play, and guided practice, 99–101
  establishing time limits for doing homework, 98–99
  overview, 11, 195–196
  reviewing homework on practice of, 106–107
Token economies. *See also* Classroom behavioral intervention; Positive reinforcement; Reinforcement; Session 5 (introducing the token economy)
  child group sessions and, 51, 59, 68, 77, 85–86, 93, 103, 111–112, 120
  developing, 82–84
  guidelines for establishing, 186–188
  introducing to parents, 82–84
  overview, 82–84, 86–87
  reviewing homework on practice of, 89–90, 97–98
Training, 32
Treatment response, 22–23, 24. *See also* Outcomes

Video-based delivery. *See* Telehealth methods
Virtual delivery. *See* Telehealth methods

Young children, 9, 129

Printed in the USA
CPSIA information can be obtained
at www.ICGtesting.com
CBHW081937240624
10583CB00004B/19